FAMILY SECRETS

Doug Dalzell

Published by Kepson Press, LLC, Kansas City, Missouri

ISBN 978-0-9849287-3-6

Cover Photos by Joshua Hoffine

Edited by Frank Kresen at Proof Positive

Dedication

To those with the courage to believe the best of people and the strength to act on their beliefs.

Chapter One

Present Day

The Tylenol PM had done its job. Jason Conrad, groggy and still half asleep, finally heard his cell phone beeping.

"Who the hell wants me at 5:30 a.m.?" he said aloud.

Looking at his phone, he saw three text messages from Dan Johnson. He dropped the phone and covered his head with the blanket. The phone beeped again.

"Go away," he yelled.

It had been a late night of drinking. His head hurt, his mouth felt dry, and he was nauseous. He felt like vomiting, but that would mean having to get up. Taking the sleep aid was a mistake, he thought to himself. Slowly, he sat up in bed. Putting his feet on the floor, he held on to the nightstand to steady himself.

"Okay, take your time. You can do this," he repeated. "One step at a time."

Looking into the mirror, he felt old. It had been four years since his wife, Alyssa, had been murdered. He still mourned her. Sleep was hard to come by. For the past three years, he'd lived in his grandfather's home. Oliver Conrad had died of a stroke just after Alyssa's murder. Jason still held him responsible for her death.

The guest quarters on the third floor were now his home. Oliver had left the 10,000-square-foot, 100-year-old mansion to him in his will. At first, Jason had been reluctant to live there. His sister Claire had finally convinced him to move in. Nothing in the house had changed since Oliver's death. For Jason, it was merely a place to sleep. Sitting on the chair next to the bed, he reached for his cell phone.

"Four texts from Dan," he mumbled. "I guess I'd better see what he wants."

The messages were brief and repetitive.

Call me!!!

"So, what's so important to interrupt my sleep?" Jason asked his former father-in-law.

"I'll be there in 30 minutes. Be ready," Dan ordered.

Dan was now his boss. After leaving medical school, Jason had enrolled in the Chicago Police Academy. Graduating high in his class, it didn't take long for him to be promoted. The work had become his passion. It gave him focus. Johnson, now second in command at the 71st precinct, had pulled strings to get Jason assigned to his unit.

It took only 15 minutes to get ready. He'd gotten used to having a three-day-old beard. He needed only a quick shower. As he looked into the mirror, he wondered what Alyssa would have thought about who he had become. The air was already thick with humidity as he sat in a chair on the front porch.

"Same chair I sat in when I had my talk with Oliver," he said aloud.

He closed his eyes and thought about the days he and Alyssa had spent there after returning from their honeymoon.

"Jason, wake up," Dan said, as he shook him.

"Dan. Sorry - just dozed off for a minute."

"What were you thinking about?" Dan asked, as he pulled up a chair.

"The time Alyssa and I spent here after the honeymoon."

"Oh. Good time, wasn't it?" Dan responded.

"Yes, a very good time, although I can't say many other memories of this house are good."

"You ever forgive Oliver?" Dan asked.

"I don't know, Dan. I guess so, but I won't ever forget what he set in motion," Jason replied. "How about you? She was your daughter."

"Jason, I'm old. Forgiveness is easier when life expectancy gets shorter. I forgave him long ago. I know that's what Alyssa would've wanted me to do."

"Yeah, you're right - she would have," Jason replied. "So, what's so important that we're getting such an early start?"

Dan shifted his weight and moved forward in his chair.

"Herman Wise called me last night. Do you remember Herman?"

"Yeah, the Wilmington Chief of Police, right?" Jason answered.

"Yep. Herman told me they have an eyewitness to the Robert Hollis murder."

"Who?"

"Leon Hingle. Apparently, he witnessed the murder. He was arrested for armed robbery in North Carolina three years ago. He's been in prison in Raleigh ever since."

"Who the hell is Leon Hingle?" Jason asked.

Dan knew who Hingle was. He had identified him and Vince D'Ambrose during his investigation of Alyssa's death. It was clear that Leon was going to give Vince up. In doing so, there was a chance he might also give up Anthony Savuzzo.

"Hingle is a strongarm for the Chicago mob. Remember when I told you about the two guys that were in Wilmington?" Dan replied. "Hingle was one."

"Oh, yeah. Who was the other one?"

"Vince D'Ambrose. He was the brains and most likely the hit man."

"There has to be more here," Jason remarked.

"There is. I think Hingle is going to turn state's evidence against Vince and his boss, Anthony Savuzzo, in exchange for witness protection and a new life."

"Will they link my grandfather to anything?"

Dan hesitated to answer. It was possible. It depended on Savuzzo. It wasn't Oliver that Dan worried about. It was James. Dan had seen Jason's father in the Chicago airport three years before when Dan was planning to go to Denver. The coincidence was hard to miss. He knew James had killed Leonard Simpson. It was the only reasonable explanation. The Simpson case was unsolved.

"I don't know, Jason. We'll just have to wait and see."

"Anything we need to do?" Jason asked.

"I contacted my boss this morning and asked permission to go to Raleigh to interview Hingle. They've isolated him to protect him against the other inmates. They don't want someone to get to him before he testifies."

"Mind if I go?"

"No, that's why I'm here. Go pack a bag. We're catching the 9:30 a.m. flight to Raleigh."

Jason hurriedly packed an overnight bag.

"You think we could drive down to Wilmington after we finish talking to Hingle?" Jason asked. "I'd like to see Kenny Conrow and Melinda Cassina."

"I was planning to do that already," Dan replied. "Have you kept in touch?"

"Yeah. We actually talk every week or so. They both took a year off to do fellowships. They graduate next May."

"It'll be good for you to see them," Dan replied.

Chapter Two

The flight to Raleigh took two hours. Wise agreed to meet them at the airport and take them to the prison that housed Hingle. He would also take them back to Wilmington to see Kenny and Melinda. It was July, and the heat was oppressive. Stepping out of the Raleigh airport felt like being hit by the exhaust from a blast furnace.

"Holy crap, it's hot here," Jason remarked.

"And humid," Dan added.

Herman waited in his car next to the exit.

"Dan, over here."

Dan and Jason hurriedly moved toward Wise's car.

"Damn, Herman - I hate July in North Carolina. Too hot and too humid," Dan stated.

"Dan, you're a pansy. This is great weather - you'll get used to it."

"Can you turn the AC up?" Jason asked from the back seat.

Herman was a tall, lanky, North Carolina native. He had been born and raised in Wilmington. It was his home. His southern accent belied his keen mind and sharp wit. He understood people.

"So, Herman, what do we have here?" Dan asked.

"Well, we have someone who wants a get-out-of-jail card and is willing to tell what he knows."

"What's he know?"

"Who killed Hollis, to start with."

"How do we know he's legit?" Jason asked.

"Because he knew about the torture. We never released that to the press. He was there. He knew exactly what happened to Hollis."

"Herman, what did happen to Hollis? All we heard was he was shot in the back of the head," Dan asked.

"He was tortured first - according to the Raleigh Police, by Hingle.

He described in detail what he did. It was exactly what we found. He was there, no doubt," Herman responded.

"Tortured?" Jason asked.

"Yes. He went through a lot before he was shot."

The trip to the state prison took 30 minutes. By the time the car had cooled down, they were pulling into the parking lot. A short walk took them to the entrance. The Warden cleared them. Within minutes, they were waiting in the visitors' area for Hingle to arrive.

"Herman, how do you want to do this?" Dan asked.

"Let's just let him tell his story. He's already talked to the FBI, so this will be a rehash."

Hingle entered and took a seat at a table in the middle of the room. Jason, Dan, and Herman took seats opposite him. Hingle was a small man. Stocky in build, he possessed huge, block-like hands and piercing eyes. If it was true that he had tortured Robert Hollis, he looked the part.

"Leon, my name's Herman Wise, I'm the Wilmington, North Carolina Chief of Police. This is Dan Johnson and Jason Conrad, of the Chicago Police Department."

"So you left medical school and became a cop. Figures - with him as your father-in-law," Hingle replied, looking at Dan.

"Have we met?" Jason asked.

"Sort of," Hingle answered. "I tailed you for a couple weeks. You never knew, did you?"

"No, I didn't."

"We stayed away from you," Hingle said, looking at Dan. "We thought you might feel the tail."

"Leon, tell us what you know," Herman asked.

"I've already been over this with the FBI, but, if you insist."

For the next 30 minutes, Hingle went over every detail of his time in Wilmington. He left nothing out. Dan and Jason sat spellbound. Everything he said checked out. It was consistent with what they had uncovered. Only

Dan knew of the connection to Anthony Savuzzo. Leon wasn't important to the FBI; Savuzzo was. Dan knew the FBI wouldn't be able to implicate Savuzzo unless D'Ambrose could be turned. Only D'Ambrose had actually spoken to Savuzzo. With Hingle's testimony, they might have the leverage to get to Savuzzo.

"Did Hollis say anything about Alyssa Conrad?" Jason asked.

"He denied killing her. When Vince was about to pop him, he looked like he recovered all the memories of the night. He actually looked content. Up until then, he only admitted that he remembered her being in his car that night," Leon answered.

"Do you know where Vince is right now?" Herman asked.

"No, but I'm sure the FBI will find him."

There wasn't anything else Hingle could tell them that they didn't already know. The FBI had taken over jurisdiction of the case. Only out of professional respect had Herman and Dan been allowed to visit.

Driving away from the prison, Dan worried that Oliver and James Conrad would be exposed. He hesitated to say anything to Jason. If Vince D'Ambrose was arrested and charged, it was possible that he would give up his boss and those connected to him.

Chapter Three

The drive to Wilmington took three hours. Jason hadn't been back since leaving three years before. Except for Kenny and Melinda, he had no reason. The memories of Wilmington were bittersweet. Herman agreed to drop them at "Tarheels" where Kenny and Melinda would pick them up. The local University hangout had been a favorite of Jason and Alyssa's. As he walked in, Jason could see his friends at the end of the bar. Kenny looked the same - tall, thin, red haired, and laid back. Melinda, as usual, was strikingly beautiful. Her long blond hair flowed over her shoulders. She was better looking than he remembered.

"Hey, bud, it's great to see you," Kenny yelled.

Melinda walked over to Jason and put her arms around him.

"Melinda, it's so good to see you."

"Ah, watch the hands, dude," Kenny remarked. "You're hugging my fiancée."

Jason stepped back.

"Why didn't you tell me?"

"Because it happened only last night," Melinda answered.

"You lucky dog," Jason said as he looked at Kenny.

Kenny smiled and pulled Melinda to him.

"Ah, you look a little haggard," Melinda said to Jason. "Got a little beard going there."

"Nah, just too lazy to shave this morning. You look amazing."

"Thank you," Melinda responded.

"And me?" Kenny asked.

"You? Well, you're one lucky son of a gun," Jason commented. "The other guys in the class must be drooling with envy."

"Yeah, I know. I'm lucky," Kenny responded. "It just happened."

"Tell me more. How'd you guys get together?"

"When you study with someone every night, you get to know them pretty well," Melinda replied. "I learned how amazing Kenny is."

They had fallen in love. The transition from study partner to lover wasn't hard. The wedding was set for three weeks after graduation.

"How're you guys going to handle residency?" Jason asked.

"We go as a package deal," Kenny replied. "Wherever Melinda gets on, I'll follow."

Kenny had finished number one in his class. He could write his ticket to any residency he desired. He chose to follow Melinda because he loved her.

"I have a feeling you'll do okay. I'm sure wherever Melinda ends up, they'll be thrilled to have you as well," Jason commented. "What are you going into?"

"I'm going into Orthopedic Surgery," Melinda replied. "Kenny's going into Cardiology."

"Wow, my dad's an Orthopod. Bill's a cardiologist," Jason remarked. "Maybe you need to come to Chicago for residency. I can put in a good word for you."

"That would be great, Jason - thanks," Melinda replied.

The thought of two of his closest friends being in Chicago excited him. Except for Jeff Dodson, the best man in his wedding, he had few friends.

"How're you doing, Jason?" Melinda asked. "What's it like being a cop?"

"I love it," Jason answered. "I think I was meant for this all along."

"Ever fire your weapon?" Kenny asked.

"Kenny, you don't ask a cop that. Don't you know better?" Melinda scolded.

"It's okay, Melinda. No, Kenny, I never have, and I hope I never will."

"So what's happening at UA?"

It had been three years. Jason had purposely not kept up with his former school. The memories weren't good.

"Wow - so much to tell you," Kenny replied.

"What happened to Gary Sherman?"

"He got fired. Last I heard, he moved back to Dallas. The local DA didn't file any charges. Treatments for Jimmy didn't work. He died a year after you left," Melinda told him.

"And the University?"

"Jasper Ogden was rehired as President. Linda Phister came back in Admissions, and they hired a new person to oversee Student Affairs."

"How about thc Board?"

"After Simpson was killed, the Vice Chair, Herbert Kraft, took over," Kenny continued.

"How about the Legacy program?" Jason asked.

"From what I can tell - and it's pretty hush-hush, the University was able to get back the money Hollis had placed in offshore accounts. Susan Hollis cooperated."

Jason wondered if Susan had been able to keep the funds her husband had transferred to her. He decided not to ask.

"Is she still in town?"

"No, she moved to Charlotte to be near her parents. She sold the beach house and the house in Wilmington. I think she just wanted to start over."

"Funny how life changes on a dime," Jason remarked. "Think of where we all were four years ago and how different life is now."

Jason loved his job. Each day was new and exciting. Dealing with the public was his forte. He didn't want to do anything else. Often, he wondered what Alyssa would've thought of him pursuing the same profession as her father. He knew in his heart she'd be happy that they were working together.

Dan had decided to leave Jason alone to visit his friends. He didn't want to intrude. He had asked Herman to drop him at the Downtown Hilton. Seeing Willie at the bar was a surprise.

"Willie, how're you doing?"

"Mr. Johnson, I'm fine. How you doing?"

"I'm good."

"I kept up with everything in the papers. Looks like you all got your man."

"Well, sort of. Actually the bad guys got them. Justice was done."

"What you doing in town?" Willie asked.

"We came down to talk to somebody in Raleigh. I brought my son-in-law down to visit some of his friends at the University."

"That's cool. Can I buy you a drink?" Willie asked.

"No, but I'd like to buy you one," Dan replied. "If not for you, we wouldn't have found out who killed my daughter."

"No, I can't let you do that," Willie responded. "I have a daughter, and I try to imagine losing her. It breaks me up."

"Well, at least give me a double, so I can give you a good tip."

Kenny agreed to give Dan and Jason a ride back to the airport. Melinda decided to come along. It was the first time Dan had seen Kenny and Melinda since leaving Wilmington.

"Hey, guys, you look great. It's so good to see you," he said as he got in the car.

"Mr. Johnson, I'm glad you came," Melinda replied.

"Dan, guess what? Melinda and Kenny are engaged," Jason remarked.

"Congratulations."

"Thanks, Mr. Johnson; it just happened last night," Melinda responded.

"Well, I can't think of two better people to be together."

Chapter Four

The last flight out of Wilmington was at 7:00 p.m. Dan and Jason barely made it, arriving at the airport at 6:15 p.m. It would be past midnight when they got back to Chicago. The visits with old friends had been worth the drive down from Raleigh. The memories of the time he'd spent at the University were still fresh in Jason's mind, as was the death of Alyssa. It was difficult driving past places where they'd shared experiences.

"I'm glad we're leaving," Jason said to Dan, as they sat at the gate waiting for their flight.

"I understand," Dan replied. "Lots of memories here, good and bad."

"Kenny and Melinda want me to come back for their graduation."

"You should. I think that would be a good thing."

"I'm surprised you didn't look up Jane Moran while you were here."

Dan smiled. He'd gone by to see her at her office.

"Well, actually I did. We had a nice visit. Don't laugh, but she's coming to Chicago in a couple weeks for a meeting of the Bar Association. We set a dinner date."

"You're funny," Jason laughed. "You weren't going to tell me, were you?"

"Why should I? It's personal."

Dan and Jane had made a connection. The chemistry was still there. Neither had found anyone else.

By the time they arrived back in Chicago, it was 1:00 a.m. The air was still heavy with humidity. It had been a hot day in Chicago, and the remainder of the week promised heat indexes of 100 degrees.

"Wow - it's still hot, and it's after midnight," Dan remarked.

"It feels like Wilmington," Jason replied.

Dan dropped Jason off at Oliver's house and drove home. Walking into his grandfather's house was always eerie for Jason. He thought often about how perfect a setting it would make for a horror movie. It was a castle. Jason had never actually been in every room. There were too many. The basement was somewhere he never ventured. As a child, he dreamed of ghosts that would attack him if he went down the stairs. Every time he walked past the door to the basement, he would pause and look around the corner, just in case. Except for Oliver's driver, Frederick, the elder Conrad had no servants. He didn't like people and chose to do what needed to be done on his own. The house showed it. Jason could recall the musty odor. Dust was everywhere. Once a month, James called a cleaning service to come in and clean his father's house. Oliver hated the intrusion but tolerated it. The darkness of night made it all that more spooky.

Jason slept hard. Tired from a long day and a short night the day before, he never heard his cell phone ring. He woke to see he had a voicemail. It was from Dan.

Jason, just calling to tell you Vince D'Ambrose was captured tonight in New York by the FBI. Herman just called me to let me know.

It was 8:00 a.m. He was late for work. Quickly he showered and dressed. The shoulder holster he put on held a standard-issue police revolver. As of yet, he hadn't used it. He hoped he never would. Walking down the hallway on the first floor, he glanced around the corner by the basement door. *Coast is clear*, he thought to himself. His car was parked behind the house. The door off the kitchen led to a mud porch and courtyard.

"Damn heat," he said aloud, as he walked to his car.

On the drive to his precinct, his phone rang.

"Jason, it's Jeff. Where you been?"

Jeff had been Jason's best man at his wedding. He was his best friend. It had been four years since a downtown brokerage firm had hired him. His ability to talk to people made him a success. With an annual income of over half a million dollars, he'd bought a downtown condo. He was living well.

"I just got back from Wilmington. Dan and I had to interview someone in Raleigh, so we took a side trip to Wilmington."

"How was it?"

"Bittersweet. It was nice seeing friends, but I have no desire to go back."

"Hey, I'm having a little get-together at my place tomorrow night. I'd like you to come," Jeff asked.

"Sure. What time?"

"8:00 p.m. Now there will be women there so are you going to be social and talk to people, or just mope around?"

"Okay, you want social, you'll get social," Jason laughed.

Jason had plenty of opportunities to date. At 6' 2", he was a handsome man. He worked hard to develop a fit body. His dark hair accented deep-blue eyes that caught the attention of young women.

"Just leave a few girls for us. It's tough for us chubby, short guys to get girls to pay attention. Okay?" Jeff chuckled.

"Jeff, women flock to you. Man you're rich, single, you have a great place to live, and, best of all, you have me as a friend."

"Hey Jason, I have an idea. Why don't we have the party at your place?"

"My place? My grandfather's house?"

"Sure. It's cool. It's huge. It's unique. It would be perfect," Jeff replied.

"I haven't cleaned anything. It's dusty, dark, and it smells old."

"Better yet. Let's do it."

"Okay, but I'm not promising anything. They may hate it."

"Everybody will love it. Besides, you have plenty of space if people want to pair up."

Chapter Five

To avoid embarrassment, Jason contacted the cleaning company that James had used in the past to come in and clean Oliver's house. Jeff hired a caterer to provide all the food and alcohol. Sitting on his porch at 7:00 p.m. the night of the party, Jason began to have misgivings.

"What have I done?" he said aloud. "This place will be a mess when this thing's over."

It was a warm evening, but comfortable. Jason had turned the air conditioning up throughout the house. Over 60 people were expected. Most, according to Jeff, were single. Jason remembered his conversation with Jeff from two days before.

"Hey dude, we don't want just old, married people here. We want some possibilities. There will be young, good-looking women doctors, lawyers, business associates, teachers, grad students - you name it," Jeff had told him.

"Just so long as they aren't part of biker gangs, okay?"

"Jason, you need to get out. It's been three years. Alyssa would want you to find someone, you know that."

Jason didn't respond. He still found it difficult to talk to women. He hadn't opened himself up to the possibility.

Jeff arrived at 7:30 p.m. He parked on the street and took a seat next to Jason on the porch.

"Caterers get here?" Jeff asked.

"Oh yeah. They're all set up. There's plenty of food and two bars. My grandfather would turn over in his grave if he saw what was happening in his house tonight."

"Jason this is your house now. You get that? It's your house."

"It's still hard to grasp," Jason replied.

"Is Claire coming? I know she's in Chicago."

"Sorry, buddy, but Claire and Jackson got married last year. I know you always had a crush on her."

"I know she got married. I just thought she might come."

"Meredith and Bill won't be here, either. I'm the only Conrad you get, unless you count the ghost in the basement," Jason laughed.

Claire Conrad, Jason's older sister, had finished her residency and taken a job in Chicago. Her husband, Jackson, followed her and was now a staff Pathologist at Cook County Hospital. Jason's brother Bill was a practicing cardiologist. Meredith, who had graduated from Harvard, was completing a residency in Internal Medicine at Barnes Hospital, in St. Louis, Missouri.

Jason met guests at the door to welcome them. Jeff was right. He had invited a very attractive, highly successful group of people. They came from every walk of life. The one thing they had in common was that they were all good looking.

"Damn, Jeff, did you have them send pictures in before you invited them?"

"Yep, I checked everybody out ahead of time. Is that bad?"

"Yes, that's horrible, but not surprising," Jason laughed.

Jeff shrugged his shoulders and smiled.

"So sue me."

Faces began to run together for Jason. Pretty people all grouped together don't stand out. No one seemed special. No one until Halie Carson arrived. Halie was a sixth-grade teacher in the Hinsdale School District. The school was only half a mile from Jason's home. She and another teacher, Jenny Holcomb, had been invited by a mutual acquaintance of Jeff's. When Jason shook her hand, he didn't want to let go.

"Hi, my name's Jason Conrad. Welcome to my home."

"Thank you for inviting us," Jenny interrupted.

Jason reluctantly gave up Halie's hand and pointed them toward the bar. Standing at the front door, he peered into the living room to see if he could see her. He couldn't. Halie was a beautiful woman. Her long red hair and green eyes caught the attention of men and women alike.

"Jeff, thanks for the invite," Jenny said as she moved next to him at the bar.

"My pleasure."

"This is Halie Carson. Halie, Jeff Dodson, one of the hosts."

"Hi, Halie, good to meet you."

"Jeff, you know much about the guy at the door?" Halie asked.

"You mean Jason?"

"Yes, Jason."

"Jason's my best friend. He's a cop in Chicago. This house was his grandfather's. He left it to him in his will. Jason's family is old money in Chicago."

"Is he attached?" Halie asked.

"No. He was married once, but his wife was murdered three years ago. Jason and Alyssa were med students in North Carolina when it happened."

"Oh, I'm so sorry. That had to be awful."

"It was. He loved her. He hasn't recovered yet. But it's time he got out into the world again. That's why I suggested having the party at his house. I was blown away that he agreed to have it here."

Jason continued to try to find Halie in the crowd. At the far side of the room, he could see her talking to Jeff.

"Did they catch whoever did it?" Halie asked.

"Sort of. Jason and Alyssa's dad, who's also a cop, went to Wilmington to find the killer. They found him, but someone else got to him first."

"I take it he decided to drop out and become a cop?"

"Yes. He loves it. It's his passion."

At 9:00 p.m., Jason decided to join the party. He'd done his job as host - now he wanted to relax. People had spread out throughout the house and into the back yard. Laughter was coming from every room. Slowly, trying not to be too obvious, Jason went room to room looking for Halie. He wanted to get to know her.

"You looking for me, I hope?" Halie asked, as she saw him approaching.

"Ah, well, ah, no. Er, yes, I guess," Jason stammered.

"Well I'm glad you found me," Halie replied. "This is a great party." Jason hadn't talked to a woman in a long time. He was rusty, out of practice. He tried to be cool. He wasn't. Halie could tell he was nervous. She liked the fact that he looked for her and that he wasn't overconfident. She was used to meeting men who had high opinions of themselves, mostly undeserved.

"Can we go out on the front porch?" she asked.

Jason was relieved. He wanted to get out of the crowd.

"Absolutely."

They moved outside and sat in Adirondack chairs in the corner of the front porch. Everyone else was either inside or out back.

"So, Jason, you're a cop?"

"Yep - hope that's not a problem."

"No, no, not at all. I'm a sixth-grade teacher."

"Really, where?" Jason asked.

"About half a mile from here, Hinsdale Elementary."

"You're kidding? I went to school there. So did my brother and sisters. I was the Conrad that got suspended all the time."

For the next two hours Jason and Halie talked. They talked about everything, except Alyssa. Halie was reluctant to bring it up, and Jason never did. He felt comfortable with her, much like he had with Alyssa.

"Would you like to go to a movie with me this weekend?" Jason asked.

"Sure, that would be nice."

"Can I pick you up at six? We can stop and get something to eat after the movie."

"That would be great," Halie replied.

"Hey, here you are," Jenny Holcomb said, as she walked out on the porch.

"Been here the last two hours," Halie replied.

"Well, it's time to go. We have school tomorrow. I need to look over my lesson plans once more."

"Okay, guess I should do that, too."

Jason hated to see her go. For the first time since Alyssa's death, he was enjoying the company of a woman. He felt excited and guilty.

"Glad you all could come. Six on Saturday. You have my number; just text me your address," Jason called out as Halie walked down the sidewalk.

"I will."

"Six on Saturday. You have a date with him?" Jenny asked.

"Actually, yes," Halie replied.

"I thought you didn't go out with guys you met at parties."

"Well, I made an exception."

"He's good looking. Is he nice?" Jenny asked.

"Very."

Chapter Six

Jason walked back inside. Jeff, as he expected, had left with a young attorney. By midnight, everyone was gone. The caterers had closed up at 11:00 p.m. Only a few diehards remained. Getting up from his grandfather's favorite chair, he surveyed the damage. Beer bottles, dirty plates, empty glasses, and other trash littered every room in the house. Walking into the kitchen, he noticed the door to the basement was ajar.

"Oh, crap. Somebody went down into the basement," Jason said aloud to himself.

He'd never been in the basement. Oliver had strictly forbidden it. Jason hadn't ever wanted to go there. Now he had to. He decided to save it for last. Closing the door, he made his way to the pantry for trash bags. Over the next hour, he went from room to room, collecting trash. Some rooms he hadn't been in since childhood.

"Damn, people can sure make a mess," he lamented.

After two hours of cleaning, all that remained was the basement. Slowly approaching the door, he felt his heart starting to beat faster.

"I'm a cop. What am I afraid of?" he asked himself.

Just for safety, he grabbed his service revolver and a flashlight from the drawer in the kitchen. Turning the knob to the door, he reached in and turned on the light. Only a single, bare light bulb lit the basement. Slowly, he proceeded down the stairs. Near the bottom, he knelt down and peered inside. It was hard to make anything out. Two more steps brought him to the basement floor - half concrete and half dirt. *Well, I may as well check this out,* he thought to himself. The basement was cluttered with old furniture, toys, tools, clothing, and boxes full of pictures. He started to look through each box.

"Hell, I'm here now. I may as well look through this stuff," he said aloud.

Each box contained hundreds and hundreds of pictures. Most were of Oliver and Miriam. Others appeared to be of James. Some were of people Jason didn't know. Suddenly, his cell phone rang. He jumped, startled by the noise.

"Hello."

"Jason, buddy. How you doing? I just wanted to see if everything was alright," Jeff asked.

"I see you left in a rush. Meet someone?"

"Well, yes - a pretty blond attorney. I think I'm in love."

"You fall in love every week," Jason responded.

"Hey, you need any help cleaning?"

"You're a day late and a dollar short, as if you didn't know," Jason replied.

"Damn, I was looking forward to helping you clean."

"Go back to your blonde. I'm sure you left her in bed to make this call."

"Yeah, I did. Sorry," Jeff answered.

Jason hung up and went back to examining the contents of boxes. After he separated the boxes and bagged the clothing, he decided to look at the furniture. Dust covered everything. Some items looked to be from the 40s, others from the 60s and 70s. He examined each item. *I think most of this needs to go to Goodwill,* he thought to himself. Again his phone beeped. He jumped in fear and reached for his weapon.

"It's a text, you idiot," he scolded himself.

Halie had sent him a text.

Just wanted to thank you for a great night. Can't sleep thinking about how much fun it was. See you Saturday night. Halie

Jason sat down on a nearby chair. He sneezed as the dust came floating upward. He smiled as he typed out a response.

Thanks for coming. You were the best thing about the party. Can't wait for Saturday night. Jason.

As he pushed "send", he thought about Alyssa. As much as he enjoyed his time with Halie and looked forward to their date on Saturday, he felt guilty. Part of him felt like he was betraying Alyssa.

"No, don't do that. She'd be the first to tell me to be happy," he said to himself.

Sitting alone in half-light, he spied a travel trunk in the corner of the room. It was vintage 1930s or 40s. He noticed it was padlocked. He pulled it out from the corner and grabbed an article of clothing to push away the dust. On the top a mailing label read "Oliver Conrad, Chicago, Illinois." He remembered a number of keys in one of the kitchen drawers. Retrieving them, he tried each one on the lock; none worked. His curiosity was piqued. He wanted to know what was in the trunk. *Why not?* he thought to himself as he reached for his service revolver. If he fired it, he'd have to report it to his precinct sergeant. He decided he'd say he saw a rat in his basement. Everyone knew he was living in an old house. It was plausible. Drawing his weapon, he positioned it six inches from the lock. Slowly he pulled the trigger. Once the smoke had cleared, he could see the lock was still intact.

"Damn it," he said to himself. "Can't even open a lock."

He knew use of his weapon again would be hard to explain. Slowly, he pushed the trunk back into the corner.

"I'll get you open. Maybe not tonight, but if I have to saw you in two I will get it done," he said aloud to himself.

It was past 2:00 a.m. He was tired and frustrated. Before leaving the basement, he walked around shining his flashlight into corners.

"Okay, any ghosts, I'm leaving now, so you can come out. Just stay down here. Deal?" he said aloud, without a reply.

Chapter Seven

The last three years hadn't been good for Jason's father, James. Unable to focus on medicine, he retired. The work ethic and personal drive he exhibited before Alyssa's murder was gone. Fourteen-hour days treating patients and doing surgery no longer interested him. His days now were spent in quiet solitude. Dan had watched him lose direction. It started the day he returned from Denver. Dan would never divulge what he knew or what he suspected. James had done what he himself planned to do. If not for his actions, Dan, or worse yet, Jason, would have given away their future to avenge Alyssa.

When Monday morning arrived and Jason reported to work Dan wanted to talk.

"Jason, how's your Dad doing?"

"Not very well."

"I know. I saw him last week. He doesn't seem like the same person."

"After Alyssa, he seemed to not care about anything anymore. It was as if it took the life out of him," Jason replied.

It had, both Jason and Dan saw it. Victoria tried to help. She didn't understand what had happened. She didn't know why he had changed.

Dan knew what James was going through. He'd seen fellow officers try to deal with having killed someone. Some recovered, some didn't. For James, it was different. It was cold-blooded murder. It could be justified. Dan had done so many times in his mind. It was still the taking of human life. It was against the oath that James had taken as a physician.

Meeting his lifelong friend Anthony Savuzzo for lunch in a private room at the Michigan Avenue Club was something James had done often. His father Oliver had never known how involved he was in the Chicago crime syndicate. James had kept him in the dark.

"Jimmy, I'm worried about you," Anthony said.

"Why? I'm fine."

"No, you aren't. Ever since you got back from Denver four years ago, you've been different."

"How so?"

"Well, let's see. You left a job you loved and a profession that you were really good at. You mope around all day without purpose. You look terrible.

You hardly ever leave the house. I could go on and on."

"Tony, I just don't think I deserve to practice medicine anymore. I violated everything that was sacred."

"Hey, I told you to leave Simpson to us. You insisted."

"I'm not blaming you. It was my decision. I pulled the trigger. I have to deal with the aftermath."

Anthony knew why James had killed Simpson. Avenging Alyssa was part of it, but protecting his son made it a decision he didn't hesitate to make. He knew Simpson's involvement in Alyssa's death would eventually come out. He couldn't risk Jason taking things into his own hands. Anthony had taken care of Robert Hollis. It was his responsibility to handle Leonard Simpson. He wouldn't let anything hurt his son's chance for a full life. Jason had suffered enough.

"I just wish I could do something to help you, Jimmy."

"Tony, you're my best friend. You're like family."

"Hey, that still doesn't deal with how we're going to bring you out of your funk."

"I'm done with medicine. I'm retired. Unfortunately, nothing else interests me."

Anthony wished he could help. He didn't know how.

"I saw Dan Johnson last week. He said Leon Hingle has implicated you in the Hollis murder. He also said Vince D'Ambrose was captured in New York. Are you worried?" James asked.

"No. The feds don't know Vince. He'll never talk. If he doesn't, they can't link me to the hit. Hingle's not enough. I never spoke to him."

"You're not worried about Vince?"

"Not for one second. Vince knows his family will be cared for. If he faces time, he'll do it without giving anyone up."

"How about Leon?"

"I hope the best for Leon. I'm not sure I'd want to be in his shoes. Once the feds figure out Leon can't give them anything, they'll cut him loose."

"No witness protection?" James asked.

"The Feds will give you witness protection if you can do something for them. Leon can't. As long as Vince is quiet, it ends."

"So, a lot rides on Vince."

"Vince will be fine. I'll be fine," Anthony assured him.

"You know, if you ever need me," James responded.

"I know that, Jimmy. I just want you healthy again. You have too much to offer to give up."

Anthony and James were like brothers. They protected each other. They would die for each other.

Jason knew nothing of his father's activities. Dan suspected the friendship but chose to look the other way. Anthony knew Dan understood the relationship he had with Jason's father. Both had formed a friendly, yet adversarial, relationship.

Leon Hingle's decision to name names had placed a burden on that friendship. Dan didn't know what Vince would do. He feared he'd give Anthony up, thereby putting both Oliver and James at risk. He wasn't privy to Anthony's relationship with D'Ambrose. He needn't have worried. Oliver's reputation and James' anonymity were safe.

"Do you think Vince will give Anthony up?" Jason asked.

"I don't know. I'm not sure he will. People close to Anthony stay loyal."

"Of course - it's that or he kills them," Jason replied.

"No, it's not that. Anthony makes those closest to him understand the meaning of loyalty. We never could get anyone close to him to testify against him. It wasn't because they feared for their life. They just loved him."

"Loved him?"

"Yes, he does things that build that feeling."

"Wow. So, how do you get to him?" Jason asked.

"The only way is from the inside. Either you plant someone early, or you create a tie that seems unbreakable to Anthony."

"Such as?"

"I wish I knew," Dan answered.

Since his trip to Denver, James had lost interest in things he ordinarily cared about. He didn't care about money anymore. He had once. He didn't care that his father, Oliver Conrad, had left him more than 50 million dollars. Money had no meaning. Jason and his brothers and sisters would eventually benefit from what Oliver and James had amassed. Oliver had left Jason his home in his will. His hope, at the time he changed his will, was that Jason and Alyssa would live there as husband and wife. Alyssa's visits had convinced him of what he needed to do. He knew she would honor the tradition and history of his and Miriam's home. Now, it was Jason's home.

Chapter Eight

The week couldn't have gone by any more slowly for Jason. He looked forward to getting to know Halie. He called her just to make sure the date was still on. Plans were to pick her up at 6:00 p.m. and go to a movie. If they had time, a quick dinner would follow. Each night, when he could sleep, he dreamed about Alyssa. Feelings of guilt kept him awake. Going out with another woman seemed disloyal. It had been three years. He still visited Alyssa's grave every few weeks. It was his routine. He took flowers and spent an hour bringing her up to date on his life. Sometimes, he'd see Dan there.

At 3:00 a.m. on Saturday morning, he sat in his favorite Adirondack chair on the porch. It was still warm out but pleasant. A gentle breeze from the south made it comfortable. It was one of the spots Jason loved. It was quiet, especially in the early morning. He could be alone to think.

"I've got to move on with my life," he said to himself. "I've got to let go of the past if I want a future. Alyssa would want me to find someone new - just as I would've wanted her to find someone if I weren't here."

At 6:00 a.m., a police siren awakened him. He'd fallen asleep in the chair.

"Damn sirens. Guess that's part of life in the city," he said aloud.

He'd started to talk to himself. It started soon after Alyssa's death. It was his way of coping. Walking into the front foyer, he looked around at what was now his home.

"Guess I'd better clean this place up. Who knows? We may end up back here tonight," he muttered.

His Saturday was clear. Nothing was on his schedule.

"Maybe today will be the start of my new life. I have a date. I may as well check out my new home," he said to himself, as he moved from one room to the next.

Each room had a particular oddity. The living room had pocket doors that hid when open. The dining room featured built-in china cabinets in the walls. The kitchen had a ceiling made of tin. Each room had 10-foot ceilings and ornate chandeliers. Oliver's den, which had a fireplace, was off the living room. Jason looked at the chair Oliver had died in and thought about his grandfather. He still couldn't bring himself to forgive him. It would take time. Sitting in the chair, he could imagine Alyssa engaged in a lively conversation, drinking lemonade that he'd made especially for her. She'd told him about how much she enjoyed visiting.

A curved staircase led to the second floor. Off the kitchen was a second, narrow staircase, meant for servant use. He remembered playing in the back stairwell as a child. Each time he passed the basement door, he turned to make sure the coast was clear. It was his routine.

"Okay, I think I can handle the basement now," he said as he opened the door and walked down the steps.

He was proud of what he'd accomplished the last time he ventured into the darkness. The trunk still sat in the corner.

"I'm going to get you open. Don't think I've forgotten you."

The second floor contained six bedrooms, each with its own bathroom. He wondered how long it had been since anyone had slept in them. The master bedroom was in the back of the house. Oliver had wanted to be close to the back stairwell. His clothes still hung in the closet. Nothing had been touched. The cleaning service that Jason had hired before the party had done a good job. Dust had occupied every surface before they came.

Jason could afford housecleaners. His grandfather had left him not only the house but also a five-million-dollar trust fund. Oliver left each of his grandchildren an equal amount. Jason, who loved being a cop, never used any of the money. He lived on his $45,000, a year, salary. The trust gave him access to the income each year from the five-million-dollar principal. Jeff managed the assets. Jason wanted nothing to do with it. They agreed that half of the income each year would be given away to not-for-profit agencies and the rest reinvested. Jason and Jeff met on New Year's Day each year to determine who would receive the funds. Jason preferred anonymity. Jeff made the gifts in the name of Oliver Conrad. Jason's name was never mentioned.

Sitting on his grandparents' bed, he was surprised at how uncomfortable it was.

"Damn, I don't think Oliver ever replaced this mattress. How did he sleep on this thing?" he asked himself. "I guess it's what you get used to."

"Okay, this is another Saturday project. I've got to give all these clothes to Goodwill. They'll need a truck considering what's in the basement."

Another stairwell led to the guest quarters on the third floor. A full living room, bedroom, kitchen, and bathroom made it the ideal place for Jason to live. It was isolated from the rest of the house. It also had memories. Alyssa and Jason had stayed there after their honeymoon. They'd made love in the same bed that Jason now slept in each night.

"I've got to do a better job keeping this place clean."

He was thankful that the house contained a laundry chute and dumb waiter. It made the stairs less cumbersome.

"This is a workout all by itself," he complained to himself.

One of the things he liked most about the third floor was the view. Oliver's house was perched on a rise. Looking out from the front of the third floor, he could see downtown Chicago. The window off the bedroom looked toward the back yard and residential streets. In the distance, he could make out Hinsdale Elementary School.

For the next four hours, Jason cleaned, did laundry, and tackled household chores as he carried on a conversation with himself. Folding the last load of laundry, he realized it was 5:00 p.m. It was time to get ready for his date.

Chapter Nine

Halie lived in an apartment by herself in Lincoln Park. She was willing to sacrifice to live in the area. She loved the activity. This was her third year as an elementary teacher. She loved what she did. Teaching was what she wanted to do since she was 10 years old.

"Hi, hope I'm not too early," Jason said, as Halie opened the door.

"No, not at all. I'm ready."

Jason felt uncomfortable. Being with a woman seemed strange and wrong.

"You look beautiful," he stammered.

"Thank you. You want to come in for a minute? Can I get you something to drink?" she asked.

"Diet Coke, if you have it?"

Jason was surprised she wasn't attached. At times he found himself staring at her. He hoped she didn't notice.

"Thanks," he said, as she handed him the drink.

"So, what are we doing tonight?" Halie asked.

"Well, if you're up for it there's a really good foreign film at the little movie theatre around the corner."

"That sounds great," she responded. "There's a good Mexican restaurant right next to it."

As soon as Jason finished his drink, they left for the movie. A car wasn't necessary since the theatre was close by. Walking toward the theatre, Jason struggled to deal with his guilt. He wanted to be with Halie but felt sadness that Alyssa was gone.

"You okay?" Halie asked.

"I'm fine - just a little nervous. I haven't gone on a date in a long time."

"Let's just relax and have fun," Halie responded.

The movie and dinner were fun. Jason wanted to hold her hand in the movie but couldn't bring himself to make the first move. Halie could feel his reluctance. She knew he was still trying to get over the loss of Alyssa.

"You know I realize how difficult this is. There's no pressure here. I'd just like to get to know you, slowly," Halie told him.

Jason felt relieved. He could relax. The pressure was gone.

"Hey, after dinner, do you want to drive over to my house? We can have a glass of wine on the front porch."

"I'd love to. The front porch is becoming our place," Halie laughed.

The drive from Lincoln Park to Hinsdale took 30 minutes. Jason felt at ease knowing he'd cleaned the house. He wasn't afraid to show any part of it, even the basement. He parked in the back and opened the car door for her.

"A gentleman, that's nice," Halie remarked.

"I give my mother credit for that. She instilled that in both my brother Bill and me."

Victoria Conrad had done a good job giving her sons an understanding of what a gentleman was.

"My mom always said a gentleman was someone who strived to make life a little bit easier for those around him."

"That's a good description. I'll remember it," Halie replied.

Jason led her through the house out to the front porch.

"I'll go get some wine. Make yourself comfortable."

"What were those boxes on the dining room table?" Halie asked.

"Old family photos. I found them in the basement."

"Can we look at them later?"

"Sure, if it won't bore you too much," he answered.

"No, it'll be fun."

"Wow, she wants to see Oliver's old pictures. I must be really boring," Jason thought to himself.

Rummaging through the refrigerator, he found a cheap bottle of white wine.

"I hope white's okay. I'll be honest - it's cheap white."

"That's fine. Anything will do," Halie laughed.

"So tell me about yourself," Jason asked.

Jason and Halie sat back in the Adirondack chairs and sipped wine. The talk at the party was about impersonal things. Now it was personal.

"Well, let's see. I was born in Davenport, Iowa. My dad is a mailman. My mom is a stay-at-home mom. I have one brother, Harry, and one sister, Hillary. Don't laugh. I know naming all your kids with the same letter is weird, but my mom thought it would be cute," Halie said, trying to avoid laughing.

"I didn't laugh," Jason replied. "Where'd you go to school?"

"I got my Bachelor's Degree at Cornell College, in Iowa, and my Master's at Iowa State. How about you?"

"DePaul, then an ill-fated year in med school in North Carolina."

Halie hesitated to ask the next question, but knew it was inevitable.

"Tell me about Alyssa. Jeff told me what happened. She sounded like an amazing woman."

"She was. I think about her every day. It's been a long three years, but I have to move on," Jason replied. "Alyssa was a rare human being. Everybody loved her. She was intelligent, warm, caring, sensitive, and beautiful. When she was killed, it was like a bright light went out. It's taken me three years to recover."

"Are you okay?"

"Yes. I think I started my life over again today. You might not realize it, but I spent all day cleaning. It's taken a while for me to accept that it's my home, but I do now."

Halie reached for his hand and squeezed.

"So, what do you like to do when you're not teaching?" Jason asked.

"Seems like I'm always either in the classroom or getting ready. I guess my biggest interest is reading. That and sitting on the beach in some distant location," she replied. "What do you like to do?"

"I'm like you. Seems like I'm always at the precinct. I don't think I have a hobby. That sounds sad, doesn't it?"

"No, not at all. We're the same. I love my job. My job's my hobby."

"What do you enjoy most - the teaching or the kids?" Jason asked.

"The kids. I can't explain it, but it's so fulfilling."

"So Halie, do you have anybody in your life?" Jason asked timidly.

"No. I dated in college, but no one stood out. Maybe I'm too particular."

"Okay, now you're pulling my leg. You're a beautiful, intelligent, educated woman. You have to have had your share of boyfriends."

"I did, but no one special. I'm not in a hurry. When it's right, I'll know."

Jason was impressed. Halie knew what she wanted in life. He wanted to see her again.

"Let's look at those pictures," Halie remarked.

"Okay, but you're going to be bored."

Jason helped Halie to her feet and led her into the dining room. They sat next to each other at the table. Slowly, they examined the pictures in each box.

"Let's divide them up into ones you can identify and ones you can't. Would that be okay?" Halie asked.

"Sure, sounds fine to me."

Most pictures were of Oliver and Miriam, or of James growing up.

"I wonder what they were thinking at that moment?" Jason questioned, as he looked at a honeymoon picture of his grandparents.

"Probably about how great life would be together," Halie answered.

In the bottom of the last box were pictures of James when he was in college. Jason stopped when he saw a picture of his father with two other male students. He recognized the young man to his father's right. It was the same man he'd seen at the Michigan Avenue Club and at Oliver's funeral.

"You okay, Jason? You look like you saw a ghost."

"I'm fine. Just thought I recognized someone."

Chapter Ten

The evening had gone as Halie had hoped.

"Will you give me a tour of your home?" she asked.

"Sure," Jason replied.

The photo had shaken him, but he didn't want anything to spoil his date. He felt for the first time in three years that he'd found someone that he could talk to.

"This is a great house. It has so much history and personality."

"Thank you. I'm just now starting to appreciate it."

Jason took his time giving Halie a tour. He wanted the time to slow down. His feelings for her grew with each minute. Leading her up the stairs, he reached down and touched her waist to help her navigate. Just touching her made him appreciate how fulfilling it was to have someone. It wasn't sexual. It was familiar. After showing her the second-floor bedrooms, he led her to the third floor.

"This is where I live," he said as they reached the third floor.

"It's perfect. A good workout too," Halie commented.

"I know. The stairs are a bear," Jason replied.

It was late. Jason knew he needed to get Halie home. As he pulled into the parking lot across from her apartment, he thought about how much fun he'd had. His feelings of satisfaction were tempered by the guilt of realizing he hadn't thought of Alyssa the entire night. He reached for her hand as he walked her to the door. They looked at each other and smiled. There wasn't a kiss at the end of the night, just a warm hug.

"Will you have dinner with me next Friday?" Jason asked as Halie opened her door.

"I'd love to."

"Seven o'clock, okay?"

"Sure."

Halie called Jenny Holcomb as soon as she sat down. She'd promised to let her know how the date had gone.

"Jenny, it's Halie."

"Okay, how'd it go? Did you like him?"

"I like him a lot. He's a really nice person," Halie replied.

"Yeah, and it doesn't hurt that he's handsome, does it?"

"No, that's a side benefit," Halie replied.

"What did you all do tonight?"

"We went to a movie and dinner. Then we went back to his house. We sat on the front porch and talked. He gave me a tour of the house, then we looked through some old photos that were stored in the basement."

"Did he kiss you goodnight?"

"Jenny, that's personal, but no. He did hold my hand, and he gave me a hug at the door."

"Are you going to see him again?"

"We're having dinner Friday night," Halie answered.

Jason had difficulty sleeping. Thoughts of Alyssa kept him awake.

"I can't believe I didn't think of her until Halie brought her name up," he said aloud.

He needed air. It had become his nightly habit to spend time on the porch. Sitting in his favorite chair, he pulled out his cell phone. It was 2:30 a.m.

"Dan, did I wake you?"

"What do you think? Yes. Anything wrong?" Dan replied.

"I went out on a date tonight. I keep thinking about how disloyal I was to Alyssa."

"Jason, Alyssa's gone. You need to move on with your life. She'd be happy to know that you went out. Stop feeling guilty."

"I can't help it. The worst part is I really enjoyed myself. I didn't think of Alyssa at all during the night."

"That's a good thing. Tell me about your date. Who is she?" Dan asked.

"Her name's Halie Carson. I met her at a party. She teaches sixth grade at the same elementary school I attended. She's really nice."

"Are you going to see her again?"

"We have a date next Friday," Jason answered.

"I'm glad. You're doing the right thing. Now, can I go back to bed?"

"Sure, sorry," Jason replied. "Hey, I almost forgot. When Halie and I were looking at old photos that I found in Oliver's basement, I thought I recognized someone. It was a picture taken when my dad was a student at DePaul. He was standing in front of what I think was the Phi Theta Fraternity house with two friends. One looked like a younger version of the guy I saw you talk to at Oliver's funeral. I'm sure it was the same guy that I saw my dad talk to when we had lunch at the Michigan Avenue Club three years ago."

"You still have the photo?" Dan asked.

"Yeah, it's in the box."

"Mind if I take a look at it?"

"Be my guest. Hey, Dan, I'm sorry I woke you up."

"Call me anytime. See you Monday," Dan said as he hung up the phone.

Anthony Savuzzo and James Conrad, college fraternity brothers and close friends, Dan thought to himself as he lay awake. That was the connection. Now he understood how James had known about Leonard Simpson. His fraternity brother had kept him informed throughout the investigation into Alyssa's murder. It started to make sense.

"It won't be long before Jason figures things out," Dan said to himself.

Sunday morning came early for Jason. He'd called his mother early in the week to see if he could join them for brunch after church. Victoria was excited that he was coming. Since Alyssa's death, he'd been to the house only a few times. Jason was concerned about his father. As he dressed, he decided to show him the picture.

"Jason, it's great to see you," Victoria said as Jason entered the front door.

"Hi, Mom. How are you?"

"I'm fine. Your father's in the den. Brunch will be ready in 20 minutes."

Jason walked into the den and sat on the couch next to his father.

"Hi, Dad; you doing okay?"

"I'm fine, Jason. How are you?"

"Okay - I went out on a date last night."

"A date. That's great. I'm glad you're going out. You need to start enjoying life," James replied. "What's her name?"

"Halie Carson. She teaches at Hinsdale Elementary."

"That's the same school you went to," James chuckled.

"Dad, you just don't seem like yourself. I can't believe you gave up medicine. You loved it," Jason remarked.

"Jason, I'm tired. I just want to have some peace and quiet for a change. Haven't I earned that?"

Jason couldn't argue with his father. He had practiced for more than 35 years. He had earned the rest. It just seemed so unlike him.

"You all can come into the dining room. The meal's ready," Victoria announced.

"Thanks, sweetheart," James replied.

Victoria had prepared her usual Sunday brunch: scrambled eggs, bacon, waffles, baked chicken, crab cakes, assorted breads, and, for dessert, an apple pie.

"Jason, what have you been up to?" Victoria asked.

"Just work, Mom, nothing unusual."

"Jason, that's not true," James stated. "Tell your mother about your date."

"You had a date?"

"Yes. Her name's Halie, and she's really nice. She's a school teacher."

"When do we get to meet her?"

"Whoa, it's a bit early for that. Let's just see how it develops," Jason replied.

"When will you see her again?" Victoria pressed.

"Friday night. Now let's stop talking about my dating life, okay?"

"Okay, just asking," Victoria said, smiling.

Jason reached into his coat pocket and pulled out the picture. He handed it to James.

"Dad, who are the two guys in this picture with you? I found it in the basement amongst a bunch of old pictures that Oliver had stored away."

James examined the picture. He knew the two young men standing beside him.

"Jason, that was more than forty years ago. I don't remember. It looks like it was taken at a fraternity party. It could've been anybody. I don't know who they are."

"The one on your left looks like a younger version of the guy you talked to three years ago when we had lunch at the Michigan Avenue Club."

"I don't see the resemblance," James responded.

"Oh well - just thought I'd ask. There's some interesting stuff in the basement. I don't think anyone's been down there in years."

James didn't like Jason prying into his life.

"I hate to eat and run, but I need to go. I have to go visit Alyssa. Thanks for the meal. It was amazing, Mom."

"Don't be a stranger - and bring Halie by, okay?" Victoria replied.

"I will."

The drive to the cemetery took 15 minutes. In the trunk of his car, Jason carried a lawn chair. He'd picked up flowers the day before. His routine was to replace the flowers he left the previous week and sit on the lawn chair to have his conversation with Alyssa.

"Hey babe, it's me. Just finished having brunch with my parents. I know, you're proud of me for going. I need to talk to you about something. I went out on a date last night. Don't get mad, but I'm lonely and she's really nice."

For the next hour, Jason explained how he felt. He wanted her to understand.

"I'll always love you, babe. I just need to move forward with my life. I hope you'll forgive me. You'll always be in my heart."

It was a hard conversation - one that he knew he had to have to move on.

Chapter Eleven

Dan Johnson had learned to live alone. The deaths of Allison and Alyssa had created a void in his life. He filled his days and nights with work. Meeting Jane Moran in Wilmington wasn't planned. Having immediate chemistry was a surprise. Since returning from his trip to North Carolina, he'd looked forward to the Bar Association meeting. Two days before she arrived, she called to see if dinner was still on.

"Hi, Dan."

"Jane, I'm glad you called. I needed to talk to you."

"I hope you're not canceling," she responded.

"No, I wouldn't do that. I just wanted to set a time and place," Dan answered.

"I'm staying at the Marriott on Michigan Avenue. What do you suggest?"

"You get here on Thursday, so what would you say to dinner Friday night at Nomi? It's a great restaurant. I'll come by at 7:00 p.m. We can walk over. It's in the Park Hyatt, which is only three blocks from the Marriott."

"That sounds like a good plan," Jane replied.

"After dinner we could get a drink at RL. They have a great little bar. It's right across the street from the Hyatt."

"Dan, it's good to be with someone who knows where to go."

"I'm just glad you're going to be here. How long will you be in town?"

"Probably five or six days. It depends on the conference," Jane answered.

"Good - then maybe I'll get to see more of you."

Sitting in the lobby of the Marriott, Dan thought of Alyssa.

"I wonder what Alyssa would think if she knew I was actually going out with Jane?" he asked himself. "I think she'd be smiling."

Coming off the elevator, Jane saw him sitting alone in a corner of the lobby. He wore a collared white shirt, navy blue sports coat, and khaki slacks. She was impressed.

"Hi, Dan," she said, holding out her hand.

"Hi, Jane, you look great."

Jane did look good. She didn't look 46 years old. Time hadn't ravaged her skin. Daily workouts had kept her trim.

"Shall we?" Dan asked.

"Yes, I'm ready," she replied.

A short walk brought them to Nomi. The evening was full of conversation. Much of it centered on the aftermath of Alyssa's death and what was happening in Jason's life. As they made their way back to the Marriott, Dan reached for her hand. She gave it to him willingly.

They were together each of the next three nights. On the final night, Jane asked him to stay with her.

"Dan, spend the night with me?" Jane asked.

Dan didn't answer. Standing at the door to her room, he reached for her. He kissed her. It had been a long time since he'd made love to a woman. The night was full of passion and desire. When he left to go to work in the morning, Jane kissed him goodbye.

"When will I see you again?" she asked.

"How about I come to Wilmington in two weeks?"

"That would be perfect."

Dan felt like he'd found a new life. As he walked into Precinct 71, he heard his phone beep. It was a text message from Jane.

I love you.

He typed a response.

Love you too.

He had someone in his life for the first time since Allison died. He felt the warmth and love that a relationship provided. Even though they'd been together for just four days, they both knew it would last.

"What are you so happy about?" Jason asked. "No, wait, I know. This was the week with Jane. I get it. So, you have a nice time?"

Dan smiled and shook his head.

"Yes. It was a very nice time."

"When will you see her again?" Jason asked.

"I'm going to Wilmington in two weeks."

"Wow - that was fast."

"Hey, we're older, we know what and who we want. Why waste time?" Dan laughed. "Any word from Herman about whether Vince D'Ambrose talked?"

"Well, since you've been otherwise occupied, I talked to Herman last night. He said he couldn't get in touch with you."

"Yeah, yeah, so what's the news?" Dan asked.

"Vince closed up. He won't give anybody up. You were right."

"Doesn't surprise me," Dan responded. "Another dead end as far as Anthony's concerned. The FBI must be getting frustrated."

Anthony Savuzzo was safe. His confidence in Vince D'Ambrose was well placed. The FBI had hit a wall. Vince would most likely be looking at life in prison. Leon Hingle would be back in the prison population. How long he'd survive was anybody's guess.

"So, do you think they've connected my grandfather to anything?" Jason asked.

"For now, no, but who knows for how long?" Dan replied.

Dan didn't say anything about James. Jason didn't need to know. It was clear that James had kept his involvement with Anthony from his son and, surprisingly, his father.

Chapter Twelve

Jason's curiosity had been piqued. He decided to spend a few nights looking at what he found in his grandfather's basement. He and Halie had divided the pictures the previous weekend. One box contained pictures of those he could identify. They offered no mystery. His time would be focused on those pictures that were of people he didn't know.

Most were of people who were posed with either his grandparents or his father. Pictures of James growing up covered a span of 20 years, from childhood through college. College pictures were sparse. The same young man who appeared in the picture taken in front of the Phi Theta house was in one other picture. Jason hesitated to show it to his father. It was clear they knew each other and that he had lied.

"Hey, did you forget me?" Halie said as Jason answered his cell phone.

Jason looked at his watch. It was 7:30 p.m. He was 30 minutes late.

"I'm sorry. I got engrossed in the pictures we sorted through last weekend. I'll be there in 20 minutes."

"That's okay. Take your time," Halie responded. "Do we need to change the reservations?"

"No, we're going to Four Degrees. It's near you. A friend of mine owns part of it, so we'll get in."

Jeff had invested in the restaurant. Investing in new dining spots was popular. Although he hadn't experienced any return as of yet, Jeff liked being catered to. As an owner, he was. Jason hurriedly showered and changed. Twenty minutes later, he was pulling up in front of Halie's apartment.

"Forgive me?" he asked as she opened the door.

"Of course."

"I couldn't drag myself away from the pictures. They're really interesting. I find myself wanting to know who all the people are."

"I'm glad. It builds tradition and heritage," Halie replied.

"I told my parents about you last Sunday."

"And?"

"My mother wants to know when you're coming to dinner," Jason laughed.

"Any time, just waiting for an invitation."

After valet parking the car, they checked in with the hostess. She'd held their reservation in deference to Jeff.

"I'm really sorry about being late," Jason apologized.

"Not a problem, Mr. Conrad. Please follow me."

A few moments later, they rounded a corner and reached their table.

"Hey, buddy. I thought you'd never get here," Jeff said, as he rose from the table.

"What are you doing here?" Jason asked.

Jeff had brought the young attorney he had met at the party at Jason's house. When the hostess called to tell him his friend had a reservation, he decided to crash the dinner.

"Well, I just thought we could all get together and have a nice evening."

Jason looked over at Halie. She was chuckling. She didn't mind that Jeff had intruded. Jason did. Her smile took the edge off.

"We'll talk later," Jason said to Jeff, as he helped Halie into the booth.

"Jason, Halie, this is Kimberly Reynolds. Kim, this is my best friend, Jason Conrad and his girlfriend, Halie Carson."

Jason was embarrassed for Halie. They'd only been on one date, hardly enough to qualify as being in a relationship.

"Nice to meet you, Kim."

"Sorry. Jeff's a bit of an odd one," Jason whispered in Halie's ear.

"Actually, Jason, I met you at your party," Kim responded.

Jason hadn't remembered. His focus that night had been on Halie.

"Yes, I remember."

Halie gently squeezed his leg. She knew he didn't recognize Kim.

"Good cover," she whispered.

The evening was full of laughter. Jeff was an entertainer. He loved making people laugh. Making people feel comfortable was his gift. It helped him as a broker. It didn't take long for people to trust him. Halie and Kim enjoyed the evening. Each sparred with Jeff. Each refused to be dominated by his personality. Jason was impressed.

When the night ended, he walked Halie to the door. Unlike their last date, he kissed her. She welcomed the kiss. It was warm and sensitive. The first kiss led to a second and a third. The energy between them was palpable. Each felt strong desire for the other.

"I better let you get inside," Jason said, as he caressed her face in his hands.

Halie didn't want to go inside.

"Okay, if I have to."

"Tomorrow night? Movie?" Jason asked.

"Absolutely," Halie replied.

Jason kissed her cheek and released her. She haltingly opened the door and stepped inside. Once inside, she leaned back against the door and took a deep breath. Jason didn't want to leave, either. All he could think about on his drive home was Halie Carson.

"I didn't think this would happen again," he said to himself.

When he got home, he stopped at the basement door.

"Tonight's the night."

Turning around, he walked out to the garage and located a hacksaw.

Chapter Thirteen

The garage was separate from the house. It was large enough to house four vehicles. Oliver's old Cadillac sat in one spot. The car had been covered by a tarp for more than 30 years. Jason had intended to move it but hadn't gotten around to it. Oliver loved his Cadillac. It was a vintage 1939 red Cadillac convertible, with leather interior.

Up against the wall was a workbench, with tools spread out on pegboards. Jason reached for the hacksaw.

"This should do it."

As he passed through the kitchen, he picked up a flashlight. In a few seconds, he was standing in front of the trunk. Slowly, he pulled it away from the wall and over to the one light in the room. He positioned it directly underneath. With all the strength he could muster, he began to saw on the lock. Halfway through, he stopped.

"Damn - this is harder than I thought it would be."

He decided to take a break. He remembered he had a couple beers in the refrigerator. The thought of them made him thirsty. Grabbing two, he went back down into the basement. An old pink armchair sat in the corner. He pulled it out. Sitting down, he quickly consumed the first beer. As he opened the second, he started to conjecture on what was in the trunk. He knew it was heavy and that it had belonged to his grandfather. It appeared to have been well traveled. In the '30s and '40s, travel trunks had been the preferred means of transporting clothing while on trips, especially ocean voyages. The decals on the trunk showed it had been overseas several times.

"I bet you used to belong to Oliver's parents - maybe even his grandparents from the looks of you," Jason said, as he carried on a conversation with the trunk.

"So, you've been a lot of places, I see. I can tell. You're well worn."

Jason's mind turned from the trunk to Halie. He thought about her kisses and the feel of her body. He looked forward to the next night. It was getting serious. On his right hand, he wore his wedding ring. He moved it off his left hand a year after Alyssa died. He promised himself it would never leave his right hand. It was after midnight. He was tired.

"Okay, you have a reprieve until tomorrow morning. I'll meet you here at 9:00 a.m. sharp - got it?" he said, not expecting a response.

Leaving the hacksaw and flashlight, he climbed the three flights of stairs to the guest quarters. Collapsing on the bed, he was asleep within minutes.

"Hello, Jason, you there?" Jeff's voice could be heard as Jason opened his phone.

"What time is it?"

"About 1:00 a.m."

"What the hell? First you crash my date. Now you wake me up in the middle of the night. I need sleep. What do you want?"

"Sorry. I was just wondering if you had a good time? Kim and I really like Halie. She's gorgeous," Jeff remarked.

"I had a great time, and, yes, she's beautiful. I'm glad you all like her. By the way, Kim's way over your head."

"Yeah, I know. She's really hot. I don't know what she sees in me, but she seems to like me."

"Well, just don't screw it up. Don't press - go slow," Jason advised.

"I will, master. Thanks for the advice," Jeff laughed.

"Now, can I go back to sleep?"

"Sure - don't mind me."

For the first time in years, Jason dreamed about someone other than Alyssa.

The next morning, he dressed in a tee shirt and old blue jeans. He anticipated getting dirty. The trunk was on his mind. He'd gotten halfway through the lock the previous night. He wanted to finish before noon.

"Good morning, old friend," he said, as he greeted the trunk. "Hope you're ready to divulge what's inside you."

Picking up the hacksaw, he began to saw at the lock. The daylight made it easier to see. The flashlight wasn't needed. Light came in through cracks in the stone foundation and filtered down from the upstairs. He could hear a lawn tractor faintly in the distance, cutting grass. Other than that, it was quiet. Only the sound of metal against metal broke the silence. Every 15 minutes he'd stop and take a break. The pink chair offered a place to rest. Diet Coke had become his morning beverage of choice and source of caffeine. He hated coffee and found tea to be tasteless. He was on his second soda when the lock finally gave. He removed the lock and tossed it aside.

"Whew, that was a workout. Let's take a break before I open you up."

As he finished his diet Coke, his thoughts turned to his grandparents.

"I bet when Oliver put you down here, you didn't realize you'd stay hidden for decades, did you?" he said to the trunk.

"Well, I'm going to bring you into the light of day."

Putting down his soda, he approached the trunk. The lid stuck. Only after continued pulls did it give way. He lifted the lid and pushed. With a sudden jerk, the top fell back. The trunk was full. On top sat the March 18, 1948 edition of *The Chicago Tribune*. Slowly he removed the papers. Underneath were several assorted toys. Under them lay neatly folded clothing, clearly of a newborn child. Under the clothing, a blanket had been folded and placed as if to divide the items in the top of the trunk from those in the bottom. Beneath the blanket was a blue plastic tarp. As he pulled the tarp back, he stopped and moved back, collapsing in the pink chair.

"Oh my God," he exclaimed aloud.

Opening his cell phone, he dialed his father's number.

"Hello," James answered. "Hello, anybody there?"

Jason paused, unable to speak.

"Dad, it's Jason - you need to come over here, right away."

"Is everything okay? Are you alright?"

"I'm okay, but I found something that you need to see."

"I'll be right over," James answered.

Jason couldn't concentrate on anything as he waited for his father to arrive. What he'd found in the trunk made him question who he was and who his grandfather was.

"Jason, what's going on?" James said, as he walked up the sidewalk to the front porch.

"Come with me."

Jason led his father down to the basement. He walked around the trunk and stopped. James stopped next to him. Jason knelt down and pulled back the blue plastic tarp. James turned pale. Wrapped in the tarp were the skeletal remains of a newborn. All that was left was bones. The trunk, arranged as if it were a coffin, had been the child's final resting place. James staggered back to the chair. His body, too heavy for his legs to hold him up, shook.

"Dad, Dad, are you alright?" Jason asked.

James didn't respond. He stared at the trunk. He couldn't speak or move. The past had started to come back.

Chapter Fourteen

Jason opened his cell phone and called his sister Claire. He was worried about his father. Sitting in the chair in the basement of his home, James hadn't spoken or moved since the discovery of the newborn remains.

"Claire, you need to come over to Oliver's house," Jason said.

"You mean your house, don't you?" Claire replied.

"Right, my house. Just get over here quickly, okay?"

Claire was alarmed. She sensed urgency in his voice.

"I'll be right there."

It took only a few minutes for Claire to arrive. The condominium that she and Jackson Morris had purchased was only five minutes from Hinsdale. Jason met her in the foyer.

"Let's go down to the basement."

Claire didn't know what to expect. She feared the worst.

"What's going on, Jason?" she asked, as they descended the stairs.

At the bottom of the stairs, she saw James, sitting in a chair, staring at the opened trunk.

"Dad, are you okay?" Claire asked.

James didn't answer.

"He's been like this ever since I opened the trunk," Jason told her.

"So what's in the trunk that would have this kind of effect?"

"Come here, Claire."

Peering into the trunk as Jason pulled back the blue tarp, Claire couldn't believe what she was seeing.

"Tell me that's not the skeletal remains of a newborn child."

"That's exactly what it is," Jason replied. "I've been trying to open the trunk for the last couple days. I finally broke through today."

"Whom does it belong to?"

Jason closed the top.

"Oh, my God, Oliver?" Claire stated, as she read the name on the top of the trunk.

"Yep, Grandfather," Jason replied. "As soon as Dad saw the remains, he collapsed in the chair and hasn't moved or said anything."

Claire ran back up the stairs and out to her car. She returned with a medical bag.

"What are you going to do?" Jason asked.

She pulled out a vial of smelling salts and broke it near James. Slowly she waved it under his nose. Seconds later he stirred.

"That will be enough, Claire. I'm alright. I'll be fine."

"You sure you're okay?" Claire asked as she took her father's pulse and checked for any visible medical problems.

"I'm fine," he replied, as he stood, moved over to the trunk, and unfolded the tarp.

Claire and Jason felt relieved.

"Jason, where'd you find this trunk?" James asked.

"It was in the far corner under some tarps, blankets, and furniture. I came down here to clean and organize and decided to try to open it. None of the keys upstairs fit. I tried firing my service revolver at it, but it failed as well. I've been sawing on the lock with a hacksaw for the last two days."

"I don't understand. Why would the remains of a newborn be in Oliver's trunk? It makes no sense," Claire said.

"Let's not jump to any conclusions, okay?" James stressed.

James had been in the basement only once growing up. Stories of the basement ghost had kept him away. Only curiosity had given him the courage, at the age of 12, to peer around the basement corner at the foot of the steps. The trunk, hidden in the corner, wasn't visible. The sound of something moving convinced him to go back upstairs. He never ventured there again.

"We need to call someone," Jason remarked.

"No, we can't - not yet," James responded.

"What do you mean? We have to."

Claire knew her father wanted to know more before the police were called in.

"Jason, maybe Dad's right. Maybe we should look into this on our own before we call anyone else."

"So, what do you want to do?" he asked.

"Let me call Jackson. We need him to look at the remains."

"Good idea, Claire," James responded.

"Maybe I should call Dan," Jason suggested.

"Jason, please give me some time. I want to figure this out," James replied.

"We can trust Dan. He's like family."

Dan was like family, but his name still wasn't Conrad. James trusted only a Conrad.

"I know, Jason, but not yet. We have to keep this quiet for a while. No one, not Bill, not your mother, no one can know. Not until we know what we're dealing with," James commented. "Is that agreed?"

Jason looked at Claire. He was reluctant to agree. He didn't like holding something back from Dan.

"I'm a cop, Dad. How can I not tell Dan?"

"Please, Jason - just give me a little time."

"You know this puts me in a tough spot, don't you?"

"We know, Jason, but it's important," Claire stressed.

Jackson Morris arrived within 15 minutes. He'd been conducting an autopsy when he got Claire's call. He knew Claire. He knew from the sound of her voice that it was important. Claire and Jason met him on the front porch.

"Jack, I've got to ask you to promise me something," Claire started.

"What?"

"That whatever you see in the next 10 minutes, you'll keep to yourself."

Jackson raised his eyebrows.

"What could be so dire that you'd want my vow of silence?"

"Do I have it?" Claire pressed.

"Okay, I promise."

Jason led them down the steps into the basement.

"Jackson, thanks for coming over," James said, as Jackson neared the trunk.

James looked at Claire. Claire nodded to assure him that Jackson had agreed to keep what he saw quiet.

"Jackson, we need your help."

James pulled back the tarp, as Jackson looked down into the trunk.

"What the hell?"

"We need you to tell us as much as you can about what happened to this child," James said.

"Wait a minute. You found the remains of a newborn in a trunk in your grandfather's basement? Shouldn't we call the police?"

"We can't, not until we know more. That's why we called you."

"So, let me get this straight - you want me to conduct an autopsy on the remains?" Jackson asked.

"Yes," James answered.

"And how does the policeman in our midst feel about this?" Jackson asked, looking at Jason.

"I'm not happy about it, but we all agreed it needs to be done."

Jackson looked at each of them and then down at the skeleton. He was reluctant to do as they asked, but felt he had no choice. He would oblige for Claire.

Chapter Fifteen

It was 2:00 p.m. on Saturday afternoon. Jackson had returned from his pathology lab with the necessary equipment to remove the baby's remains from the trunk. As Jason watched, Jackson took pictures of the remains and meticulously removed each bone.

"Hello," Jason answered as he opened his cell phone.

"Jason, it's Halie; we still on for tonight?"

"Yeah, sure, I'll pick you up at 6:00 p.m. Is that okay?"

"You okay? You sound different," Halie commented.

"No, I'm fine - just getting some things done before I get ready."

"Okay, then I'll see you at 6:00 p.m."

Claire couldn't help hearing the conversation. Although she watched intently as Jackson did his job, she could hear what Jason was saying.

"Jason, you seeing someone?"

"Yes. This will be our third date."

"That's great. Is she nice?"

"She's great, Claire. I didn't think this could happen again, but I really like her."

"I'm happy for you," Claire said, as she squeezed his arm. "What's her name?"

"Halie Carson. We're going to a movie tonight."

"Maybe, sometime, you all could join us for dinner. How does that sound?" Claire asked.

"You sound like Mom. I'm sure Halie would like that."

"I'm done here. I think I have what I need," Jackson said as he removed his gloves.

"Thanks, Jackson. How long before you can tell us anything?" James asked.

"I should be able to give you a report in a couple days. I won't be able to tell you whose child it was, but I should be able to determine the cause of death and age of the child."

"That's a start. It'll help," James replied. "Jason, we need you to start looking into whose child it might have been. Find the truth, no matter what it is and who it might hurt."

"I will, but it's going to be hard keeping this from Dan."

"Just do your best. If you need to tell Dan, and you have no choice, then do it. I trust your judgment. If you do, please let me know."

"I will."

Jackson gathered his materials and equipment and headed up the stairs.

"Thanks, sweetheart," Claire said, as she kissed him goodbye.

"You owe me. Tonight, our place, special - got it?" Jackson laughed.

"Count on it," she replied.

James and Jason closed the trunk, covered it with blankets, and pushed it back into the corner. As they stood in the middle of the basement, they all thought about the same thing. Could this be Oliver's child? The silence was deafening.

"I feel like you could hear a pin drop in here," Claire remarked.

"Yeah, I know. I wish I'd never opened the damned thing," Jason answered.

"Let's go upstairs and talk for a while," James replied.

Jason turned off the basement light and followed Claire and James upstairs into the main parlor of the house.

"I know we're all wondering the same thing. Is this Grandfather's child?" Jason said.

"Well, let's see. It was in Oliver's trunk, and it was in the basement of his house. That's a pretty strong indication that it is," Claire responded.

"Jason, you said you found several boxes of pictures in the basement, right?" James asked. "Let's start by looking at those pictures. It might give us a clue."

"Dad, do you remember anything from your past that would tell us anything?"

"No, not that I recall, but maybe the pictures will trigger something."

"Can we meet here in the morning and begin to look into this? I need to get ready to go pick up Halie."

"Sure. Why don't we load the pictures you found into my car, and I'll look at them tonight. That agreeable with you two?" James asked.

Claire and Jason looked at each other and then back at James.

"Fine with us," Claire answered.

By the time James and Claire left, it was 4:30 p.m. Jason had 30 minutes before he needed to get ready for his date. He decided to sit out on the front porch and think about the meaning of the last six hours. Walking through the kitchen, he grabbed a beer and headed to the Adirondack chair that had become his primary place of meditation. As he passed the door to the basement, he could hear his grandfather's voice telling him to stay out. Now he knew why.

"Granddad, you had more secrets than anyone could have imagined," he said as he started a conversation with himself. "There's no way that Miriam could have known. No way. This baby can't be theirs."

It wasn't long before he'd fallen asleep. The beep of his phone woke him. Dan had texted him.

How's weekend going? You and Halie doing okay? Hope so.

Jason responded.

Date last night, date tonight. Going well. How about you and Jane?

Dan smiled. He was enjoying texting.

Glad. Jane's picking me up at airport in Wilmington next Friday.

Texting had become a regular form of communication between Dan and Jason. Alyssa had introduced it to her father before she died. The hope was that it would always keep them in touch while she was in medical school in North Carolina. Now it kept Dan in touch with Jason.

Halie opened the door just as Jason was about to ring the doorbell. It was a cool evening. She wanted to get fresh air into her apartment. An early morning storm had blown out all the humidity in the area. It was cool, dry, and calm in Chicago.

"Wow - you must have ESP," Jason commented.

"No, just getting some fresh air. It's beautiful out tonight."

"Yes, it is," Jason responded. "Do you mind if we just rent a movie on pay per view and call out for a pizza?"

Jason wasn't in the mood for an evening out. Too much was on his mind. What he needed was a quiet evening with Halie.

"Sure. I could tell when I talked to you on the phone that you had something on your mind," Halie replied. "Do you want to cancel tonight?"

"No. I need to be with you. It was a messed-up day."

"I'm sorry. Is there anything I can do?"

"No, I'll be okay,"

Halie reached out for Jason's hand and led him into the living room.

"Pick a movie, and I'll call for pizza. What do you like?"

"Pepperoni – really, I'll eat anything."

Jason sat on the couch and began scrolling the television for movies. He found a light romantic comedy and pushed the select button.

"I found one; probably take about 10 minutes to get through the previews," he called out.

Halie called a local pizza restaurant that delivered. She rounded the corner to the living room and saw Jason watching previews.

"That's great. I haven't seen that," she said, as she saw what he selected."

Jason thought to himself how accommodating she was. She was dressed to go out, yet she had no qualms about staying in.

"Hey, I hate to change plans on you. You look amazing."

Halie had dressed for the occasion. She'd spent two hours getting ready. What she finally chose to wear was her fourth outfit that she'd tried on. Her short skirt, high heels, and white cotton blouse gave her a fresh, inviting look.

"Thank you, Jason. I just picked something out of the closet. It didn't take very long to get ready."

Jason knew otherwise. He had two sisters. He knew how much time they took to get ready for a date.

The evening was relaxed and comfortable. For the next two hours, they ate pizza and drank wine at the coffee table while watching a movie. Toward the end of the movie, Halie settled into Jason's arms. The first kiss was gentle and unexpected, but it was clear they both longed for more. The second, third, and many more that followed were intense and passionate. No words were spoken as they melded together on the couch.

"Let's go into the bedroom. I think we'll be much more comfortable there. Is that alright?" Halie asked.

"Sure," Jason replied.

Falling into each other's arms on the bed seemed natural. Thoughts of Alyssa never entered Jason's mind. Making love to Halie was all he could think about. The feel of her hands touching his skin gave him goose bumps. By the time they woke, it was past 1:00 a.m. They'd fallen asleep in each other's arms after making love.

"I need to go, sweetheart. I had a wonderful night. Can I see you on Wednesday night?" Jason whispered.

"Sure," Halie replied.

"I'm going to ask my sister Claire and her husband Jackson if they'll join us for dinner sometime. Is that alright?"

"Can we make it an early dinner?" Halie requested.

"No problem," Jason replied, as he kissed her on the forehead.

Jason smiled as he pulled his car into his garage. Just as he began to close the garage door, Oliver's car caught his eye.

"I think it's time to see what's under that tarp," he said aloud.

Since Oliver's death, the car had remained covered. Jason didn't remember ever seeing the car outside of the garage. His grandfather had stopped working on it in the '70s. Turning on the overhead lights, he moved to one end of the car and untied the cords that secured the tarp. The rope was old and tight. It took a few minutes to loosen each knot before they could be removed. Slowly he began to pull the tarp, folding it as he went along.

"Wow!" he exclaimed, as he caught sight of the chrome and metal vehicle.

With a final pull, the cover was removed. He stood back away from the car.

"Damn, I didn't know it was a convertible," he said to himself.

The tarp had protected Oliver's prize possession for more than 50 years. Even though the car had lost some of its shine and luster, it was clearly a vintage automobile. Jason knew his grandfather must have taken great pride in it.

"I think I'm going to make you run again. You deserve to feel the sunshine on your hood."

Chapter Sixteen

July 1952

"Oliver, dinner's ready. Come inside," Miriam called out.

"I will - just a second," Oliver responded.

A 1939 Cadillac convertible was the focus of his attention. He loved tinkering with cars. The Cadillac was his pride and joy. He kept it covered up in the garage unless he planned to take it out or work on it. It was 1952. James was two years old. Dwight Eisenhower had just been elected President. The cold war with the Soviet Union was intense. The fear of nuclear warfare was real.

Oliver and Miriam Conrad had gotten married three years before. A year later, James was born. Oliver was 29 years old. He was a handsome, black-haired man, with deep blue eyes and an engaging smile. He was outgoing and gregarious, yet, in some ways, he was secretive and aloof. As a physician, he commanded a high salary at Cook County General Hospital. Neuro-surgeons were scarce. He was one of the best. As much as he liked his chosen profession, he liked the money it brought even more.

He had met Miriam at a movie theatre. She was taking tickets. On a dare from friends, he asked her out. To his surprise, she accepted. A short courtship led to marriage. It had taken him years to settle down and find a mate.

Making his fortune in the tool and die industry, Oliver's father, Eli Conrad, had been a larger than life character. He was known around Chicago as a powerful and ruthless businessman. His wife, Lucille, had died giving birth to Oliver. Eli never remarried, choosing instead to concentrate on business. Servants cared for Oliver. Growing up, Oliver had built attachments to his caregivers. Eli preferred to employ those who could care for his son rather than do it himself. He never felt close to Oliver and rarely showed him affection.

Eli died in an auto accident in 1945, leaving Oliver alone in the 10,000-square-foot stone mansion. At 22 years of age, he inherited the mansion and tool and die business. For four years before meeting and marrying Miriam, he enjoyed the single life and what Eli's fortune could provide. The Conrad mansion became known as the spot to be if you were young, single, attractive, and looking for a one-night stand. Women came and went on a nightly basis. Servants looked the other way. Everything changed when he met Miriam. Now it was home to both him and his young family, Miriam and James.

"James, go inside," Oliver directed.

James straggled into the kitchen and stood beside his mother, as she prepared dinner. It was a happy home, one full of love and respect.

"Ollie, dinner's ready," Miriam called out for the second time. "You have a phone call."

This car's amazing, Oliver thought to himself as he pulled the tarp up to cover it. The car was cherry red with chrome hubcaps and fenders, with a black leather interior and equipped with adjustable seats and mirrors. Miriam handed him the phone as he walked in the back door.

"Ollie, it's Al - can you come over?" Alphonso Savuzzo asked.

When Alphonso asked, it wasn't a request. It was an order.

"Sure. I can be there in 15 minutes."

"Bring your medical bag, and, if you have some morphine, bring it," he directed.

Oliver wondered what Al had planned. He had a bad feeling. The Savuzzo home was in Hinsdale, just six blocks south of the Conrad home.

"I've got to run a quick errand, Miriam. It shouldn't take long. Go ahead and start dinner without me."

Miriam had gotten used to Oliver leaving in the middle of a meal. His call schedule required his absence at odd hours of the day and night.

Oliver picked up the keys to his 1951 Ford Custom Victoria and headed south. As he drove, he thought about his father. Eli had worked hard to build his business and create something of value for his family. Oliver had lost it all through negligence and disinterest. What he hadn't known, until his father's death, was that the Chicago crime syndicate had helped make Eli successful. He recalled his first conversation with Lou Savuzzo after Eli's death. Lou was the head of the syndicate that controlled his father's business. It was a cool fall day in Chicago when Eli Conrad was buried. World War II had just ended.

October 1945

"Oliver, my name's Lou Savuzzo. I was a friend of your father's," the large, barrel chested man said as he walked away from the gravesite.

Oliver stopped and turned toward Savuzzo.

"You knew my dad?" he asked.

"Yes. He and I were business partners in his tool and die business."

"Really? I didn't know he had any partners."

"I was a silent partner," Lou replied, smiling.

Eli hadn't come from wealth. He'd worked as a manager in the office at the tool and die business. In 1935, it began to fail. When he had the chance to buy the business, Savuzzo was there to provide the funding. They met at a local restaurant and talked about Eli's belief in the potential of the business. Six months later, funds were made available for Eli to buy out the current owners.

"I really don't know what you're talking about. My father owned the business. He didn't have any partners," Oliver sternly pointed out.

Lou smiled and put his arm around him. Two men dressed in suits stood ominously on each side of them. A long black limo with the back door open sat at the side of the road.

"Let's go over to my car and have a chat."

Oliver didn't feel as if he could refuse. He didn't know who the man was or what he wanted, but he wasn't in a position to object. As Oliver and Lou got in, one of the men closed the door. Each took up a position beside the car.

"What's this about?" Oliver asked.

"Want a cigar? Eli loved these."

"No thanks," Oliver replied, as Lou lit a long Cuban.

Smoke began to fill the back of the car. Oliver coughed and asked if they could have some air.

Those who had gathered for the burial had all left. The funeral, held at the local funeral home, had been small, and only a dozen or so mourners had shown up at the cemetery.

"We own part of your company. It's that simple. We helped your dad buy the business in exchange for part of the profit. This is how it works. Each month you put $5,000 in cash in a plain white envelope and leave it at Barone's Pharmacy with the owner," Lou directed.

"Are you kidding? This sounds like extortion," Oliver replied.

"No, it's not extortion. We're partners."

"And what if I refuse?"

"You won't. Not if you value your loved ones," Lou said, smiling.

Three months after his father's funeral and his first conversation with Lou, Oliver met Lou's son Al. The payments that were due at Barone's hadn't been made. Oliver hadn't taken Lou seriously.

"Get in the car," Al said, as the black Cadillac Eldorado pulled up next to Oliver as he removed the newspaper from his mailbox.

Al was the same age as Oliver. He was Lou's heir apparent. He had two children, Maria, 10, and Celia, 8. Al had complete authority unless Lou vetoed him. Oliver continued to walk back toward his home. From behind a clump of trees, in the front yard, Bruno Caseo stepped out holding a pistol. Caseo was a block of a man. Square jawed and broad shouldered, he stood more than six feet tall. He commanded attention.

"Mr. Savuzzo asked nicely. Get in the car!" Bruno ordered.

Oliver complied. Al bent forward and grabbed him by the collar.

"Hi, Doc. My name's Al, Al Savuzzo. Where's my payment?"

"I'm not going to pay you anything," Oliver replied.

"Didn't my father make it clear that we're partners?"

"We're not partners."

"What's that car you're driving over there?" Al asked.

"A 1945 Ford Super Deluxe, why?"

"Nice car - you must be proud of it. Watch," Al said, as he pointed toward the car sitting by the house.

At that moment Caseo poured gasoline over the length of the vehicle. With a nod from Al, he struck a match and tossed it onto the car.

"No, stop! What are you doing?"

"That, Dr. Conrad, is a sample of what I will do to you, everything you own, or anyone you love, if you ever miss a payment again. Understand?"

"I understand," Oliver replied.

"Now get out of my car. Go call the fire department before your house burns down."

Bruno opened the door and threw Oliver to the ground. Al's car drove away as Oliver ran into the house to call for help. Just as he got to the front door, the car exploded. Burning metal flew into the yard and against the house. Thankfully, the Hinsdale Fire Department arrived within minutes. It was clear that Al had called in the fire alarm before he ordered Bruno to set the car on fire.

Oliver never missed another payment.

Chapter Seventeen

July 1952

Oliver was met by two menacing large men carrying weapons as he drove through the gate at the Savuzzo mansion.

"Hey, Doc, come on in," one said, as he opened the gate.

"Thanks, Bruno. How's the shoulder?" Oliver asked.

"Pretty good. Only hurts when it rains."

"Then tell Al to make you work only on dry days."

The Savuzzo mansion was more of a fortress than a home. Three separate brick houses, each nearly as big as the Conrad home, bordered a central driveway. Men stood at each corner of the grounds. It was clear no one gained entry unless they had permission. Oliver knocked as an armed man opened the door.

"Hey, Doc, this way," he instructed.

"Thanks Lenny."

The main house was more than 100 years old. The walls inside were dark cherry wood, and ornate drapes covered the windows. To Oliver, it looked like a house out of the '20s. He'd been there numerous times. Since his father's death in 1945, he'd become an important part of the Savuzzo organization. He didn't need any demonstrations to convince him to cooperate. He liked the money. It allowed him to live the lifestyle he desired.

Walking into the living room, he saw Al, smoking a cigar in front of the fireplace.

"Doc, come over here. Want a cigar?"

"No thanks. Miriam's holding dinner for me. What's up?"

"How's married life? James doing well?"

"It's great. Miriam and James are fine. How's Anthony?"

Anthony Savuzzo, two years old, was the same age as James.

"He's great."

"How's Lou?"

"Not too well, I'm afraid. The heart doctor says his infraction ratio is down to 14%. They say he could die at any minute."

"I'm sorry, Al. I wish there were something I could do."

"There is; that's why you're here. My father wants to die but knows he'll go to hell if he kills himself," Al continued. "I want you to give him a shot that will speed up the process."

"I can't do that. It's murder."

"No, it's not, and yes, you will do it," Al responded. "My father wants to die. He's in pain. You're going to help relieve that pain."

"Do I have a choice?"

"No, just do it," Al replied.

Oliver reached into his medical bag and pulled out a vial of morphine and a syringe.

"Will he feel any pain?" Al asked.

"No, he won't feel anything," Oliver answered.

Oliver hesitated. He knew that administering the drug would violate his Hippocratic Oath. Refusing to end Lou's life would cost him the life of a loved one. He had no choice. He paused for a moment and put the vial and syringe back into his bag.

"You want to be with him when I do this?"

"Yeah. Let's go," Al instructed.

Al and Oliver climbed a flight of stairs to reach Lou's bedroom. Oliver's senses became keen as he heard every step creak. He could feel his heart rate climb. He began to sweat. His hands shook. Looking around, he could see the carved heads of gargoyles that adorned the windows, doors, and railings. It was a dark house, one filled with fear and anger. Lou lay asleep in his bed. Mild sedatives had made him groggy. Oliver set his bag down on one side of the bed and moved over to the opposite side. Al stood next to the bed. Lou looked helpless. He wasn't the hulk of a man who had first approached him at Eli's funeral seven years before. A weak heart had slowly withered his body.

"You sure you want this done?" Oliver asked, looking up at Al.

"Yes. It's his time. He doesn't want to be here anymore."

"Okay. See that vial and syringe inside my bag?"

"Yeah. Is that what you're going to use?" Al asked.

"Yes. Bring it to me, please."

Al reached down and pulled out the vial of morphine and syringe. He handed it to Oliver. Oliver pulled on surgical gloves and took the vial and syringe from Al. Slowly, he inserted the syringe into the vial and extracted a lethal dosage.

"How long will it take?"

"Not long, his heart will stop soon after the morphine's injected," Oliver answered.

Al nodded his head. Oliver pulled up the sleeve of Lou's pajamas and inserted the needle. The fluid drained into Lou's vein. Within 30 seconds, his breathing stopped. Al stood silent over his father. He showed no emotion.

"Can I go?" Oliver asked.

"Yeah. You can go. Thanks."

Turning toward the door Oliver took three steps before Al ordered him to stop.

"This never gets out of this room. Understand?"

"It won't," Oliver answered.

Chapter Eighteen

By the time Oliver returned home, Miriam was busy washing dishes. She had held dinner for as long as she could. James had gotten restless and wanted to eat.

"Hi, Miriam. Is James asleep?"

"Yes. He was hungry, so I let him eat. Now he's in bed," she replied. "I have a plate for you in the refrigerator."

"Sit down with me while I eat, please?"

"Sure," she replied.

Oliver took his plate and sat at the kitchen table. He'd eaten in the kitchen with Miriam numerous times in the past. He watched as she moved around the kitchen sink, washing, drying, and placing dishes in the cupboard. *She's more beautiful today than ever,* he thought to himself.

Miriam walked over to him and sat on his lap. She stroked his hair as she kissed him softly.

"Hey, I missed you," she whispered in his ear.

Oliver pulled her closer.

"Do you know how much you changed my life?" he asked.

"For the better, I hope."

"Totally. I was sitting here thinking about how lost I was after my father died. I wasn't really in control. I am now, thanks to you and James."

"Thanks, sweetheart - that was nice," Miriam said as she kissed him again, this time with more passion.

Just as they finished the kiss they heard footsteps coming down the back stairwell. They could make out the voice of James. He was playing an imaginary game. The stairwell was in a castle occupied by the fair princess Alexandra. James rarely saw any other children. He made up his own games and his own world to entertain himself.

"Hey, James, let's go out on the front porch, okay?" Oliver suggested.

"It's a nice night."

"Good ploy to get him out of the kitchen," Miriam laughed.

As they neared the basement door, Oliver put out his hands to stop them.

"Okay, let's look around to see if the basement ghost is out. Miriam, you look left; James look right; I'll look straight ahead," Oliver said, barely able to contain a laugh.

Miriam and James stopped. They peered to the left and the right, hoping not to see the ghost.

"Always look when you pass the basement door to make sure the door is closed. Look around to be sure the ghost hasn't escaped," Oliver whispered.

"Have you ever seen the ghost?" Miriam asked.

"Only once. When I was a boy, my father told me never to go into the basement, but I disobeyed. When I got down to the bottom, I could see a figure against the wall behind a trunk. It moved. I knew it was the ghost. It had to be. I ran upstairs, closed the door, and never went down again."

"Oliver, stop scaring us," Miriam scolded.

"Okay, but I'm just trying to warn you."

James didn't say anything. He really didn't understand. All he was sure of was that his mother was frightened.

It was the turn of the decade. The American economy was thriving. After two lengthy wars, America was building again. New skyscrapers were dotting the landscape. Television was becoming the focus of the family living room, and new conveniences were making life much easier. The Conrad family settled into a routine. Miriam took care of the home and James, while Oliver took care of the family's financial needs.

Years of late-night parties and irresponsibility were gone. Oliver focused on family and stability. Balancing his medical practice with his real estate business was difficult. The Savuzzo family required constant attention. What spare time he had, he gave to Miriam and James. It was 1952, and

Miriam understood her role. She took what Oliver could give. She made her son the center of her life. They were happy. They were living the happiest days of their lives. Arguments were rare. When they happened, it was usually over Oliver's having to respond in the middle of the night to either a hospital call or Al Savuzzo.

Oliver and Miriam sat on the porch, watching James play. Miriam could tell something had happened. Oliver was distant. His attempts to interact with James were stiff and forced. She watched and wondered. Oliver knew he'd crossed a line that had to be re-established. *What I did was justifiable*, he thought to himself. He was protecting his family. Lou was old and would die soon.

"Oliver, you're not all here tonight. What's wrong?"

"I'm just tired. It was a long day."

"We appreciate what you do for us, sweetheart."

"Hey that's my job - to provide," Oliver replied.

"It's not a job. It's a life."

"I know. That's what I meant. It's fun watching James grow up," Oliver responded, wanting to change the subject.

"Yes, it is. Someday, he'll be like his dad."

Watching James play, Oliver thought about how he had been with his father, Eli. Work, for Eli, had been his life. Oliver rarely saw his father. He had no male role model to emulate. He always wondered if Eli had blamed him for his mother's death. It was as if looking at Oliver was a reminder that she had died because he'd been born. Rather than interact and be a father he chose to withdraw into work. Growing up in Eli's house wasn't easy.

Thanks to his father, Oliver was now in something that he couldn't control. Al's call had brought apprehension. It was that way every time any of the Savuzzo's contacted him. He lived his life in fear. *Something has to change*, he thought to himself. He remembered the feeling he had the first time Al Savuzzo called and asked him to come to the Savuzzo compound. It was early in 1947.

Chapter Nineteen

July 1947

It took only one threat for Oliver to fall in line. It was clear to him that the consequences of refusal were severe. More than a year had passed since Eli's death. Payments to Lou were now timely. When he lived up to his part of the partnership, he was left alone, left alone to enjoy his life. It all changed when Bruno Caseo was shot in a dispute with a rival at a local bar.

"Oliver," it's Al. "Get over here, now!"

"What's wrong? I'm not late. What did I do?" Oliver asked.

"Nothing. Just get over here and bring your medical bag."

The drive to Al's took only 10 minutes. Oliver drifted between fear, anger, and apprehension. Al Savuzzo was a man to fear. Waved inside by waiting guards, he parked and ran toward the door. Lenny Viglio opened the door and pointed to an upstairs bedroom.

"They're upstairs."

Oliver climbed the stairs and entered one of the second-floor bedrooms. Lying on the bed was Caseo, with a gunshot wound to his shoulder.

"What happened?" Oliver asked.

"Family dispute," Al replied.

Oliver moved over to the bed and examined the wound. It bled heavily, but wasn't fatal.

"Al, I'm just an intern. I don't think I can do this," Oliver stated.

"Do it," Al yelled

"This will take some time so if you don't mind I'd like some privacy?"

Al and his men exited, leaving Oliver alone with his patient. An hour later, he'd removed the bullet and closed the wound. A painkiller helped

Caseo get to sleep.

"Hey, Doc, thanks. Someday, I'll pay you back. I keep my promises," Bruno whispered as he fell asleep.

"He'll be fine. It was a clean wound. It didn't hit anything," Oliver reported.

"Great. I appreciate you coming over," Al replied from his favorite chair.

"It's alright. Scared me, though. I thought I was in trouble."

"Tell you what. You come when I call, when I need you, and I'll throw some information your way that might help you make it big. Deal?"

Oliver didn't hesitate.

"Deal."

Returning home, he realized he'd made a decision that would affect his life forever. He decided to be there when Lou and Al needed him. He had no doubts that they would help him secure the wealth he desired. As he sat at his desk, waiting for friends to arrive for a dinner party, he thought about what his relationship with the Savuzzo family meant. He needed them if he was to secure independent wealth. The day before his visit to treat Caseo, Harry Marcus, General Manager of the tool and die business, had called him.

"Dr. Conrad, this is Harry Marcus. I'm the GM at the...." he started.

"I know who you are, Harry. What do you need?"

"I hate to say this, but we're in real trouble."

Oliver paid little attention to his father's business. He'd used it to drain cash for his lifestyle leaving the business in peril.

"What do you mean?"

"What I mean is our sales are down. The unions are making threats. We have very little operating cash, and our creditors are at our throats."

Without constant supervision the tool and die business that Eli had built was slowly dying. The economic conditions in the United States, the War, and the move to mechanized factories had dealt a death blow to the

Conrad Tool and Die.

Lou Savuzzo anticipated that Oliver would let the business die. He knew people. He knew that Eli Conrad's son didn't have it in him to be a successful businessman.

"Al, Oliver's going to let the business die. I know it. I can feel it. He's no Eli," Lou told his son.

"So what do you want to do about it?" Al asked.

"Let it die. I think it's burned out, anyway. I don't think it would matter if Eli were here or not."

"And Oliver?"

"We need him. Let's bring him in. We can use him. Seems like somebody in our organization is always getting shot or hurt. Let's make him our Doc," Lou replied. "We'll give him some tips on available real estate in Chicago. If he makes something happen, we'll take a percentage."

"How about the $5,000 a month he's paying us?" Al asked.

"That continues. If the business closes, he'll have to find somewhere else to get the money. Hell, he's a doctor. He can come up with it somehow," Lou laughed, as he lit a cigar.

Al got up to leave.

"Where you going?" Lou asked.

"Oliver's got another party tonight. I'm going to get ready."

"You like his parties, don't you?"

"Yeah, he knows how to throw a party. You should see the women that are there."

Fifty to sixty friends were due to arrive within the hour. As usual, Laynie Jessup had prepared food for the group. Laynie was the Conrads' housekeeper. She'd been Oliver's father's housekeeper before him. Oliver and Laynie had a special relationship. It was more than just employer and employee. The years they'd spent together in the Conrad home had made them close. She cleaned and cooked all day to ensure that everyone was well cared for. She was used to Oliver's parties. Liquor flowed, and, by the end of the night, the only thing she could be sure of was that each of the Conrad bedrooms would be occupied. The only question was by whom.

"Oliver, can you ask your guests not to use the kitchen sink as a toilet?" Laynie asked.

"Laynie, no one uses the sink."

"Yes they do," Laynie said, with an edge to her voice. "I don't mind getting everything ready for you all, but I deserve a little respect. You and your friends get drunk at every party. Have some class, and don't make an ass out of yourself."

Laynie had never been so blunt. She'd had enough. The weekly parties had pushed her to the edge.

"I'm sorry, Laynie. I'll try to reel them in tonight. You don't deserve to have to put up with our misbehavior."

"I'm not judging you, Oliver. You're free to do whatever you want in your home. I just think you're heading for real unhappiness if you don't get control of your life. You're a wonderful man, and you deserve the best," Laynie remarked.

At that moment, Oliver felt close to Laynie. He reached out and drew her into his arms.

"Laynie, I'm so sorry. You're the last person I want to let down."

"I know, Oliver. We've been together for a long time. You've been a part of my life for as long as I can remember."

She didn't want him to let go. The feelings that she had for him were far deeper and emotional than either had realized.

Chapter Twenty

Laynie was 28 years old. She lived in the guest quarters on the third floor of the Conrad home. For the past 12 years, she'd served the Conrad family. Eli hired her when she was 16. Oliver, at the time, was 12. Her duties focused mainly on housekeeping. Keeping up with the Conrad mansion was no small task. Oliver had known Laynie for most of his life. She was witness to everything that went on in the Conrad home. She was there to see Oliver grow through his teen-age years, go off to college, and, finally, medical school. She was there when Eli died and when Al Savuzzo set Oliver's car on fire. She was a beautiful woman, with striking features. Her long black hair was pulled up in a bun. Her smooth, dark complexion never carried any make-up. It didn't need to.

"Oliver, you're going to get that car hit, parking it on the street," she remarked.

"If I do Laynie, I'll just get another one."

Things were going well for Oliver. Even though the tool and die business had been going badly, several real estate opportunities that Lou Savuzzo had directed him toward had become extremely profitable. The $5,000-a-month payments to the Savuzzo family hadn't been an issue. Between his salary as an intern and the profit from the real estate deals, Oliver was comfortable. It had been two years since his father Eli had died.

"Laynie, can you make sure everything is ready for tonight? I want this party to go well," Oliver instructed.

Another Conrad bash, Laynie thought to herself. *The cleanup would take all of the next day.*

"Sure, Oliver - everything will be perfect."

To be invited to a Conrad party was an achievement. Many from Chicago wanted the invitation. Few received it. Oliver's parties, held usually on Saturday nights, started slowly - only a dozen or so people, mostly close friends. Crowds grew as word spread of the lavish layouts of food and alcohol. As more and more attractive young women came, more demand grew for invitations. Even Al Savuzzo had asked to be invited. Now, he was a regular.

People started to arrive at 8:00 p.m. It was fashionable to be late. Many came between 10:00 p.m. and 11:00 p.m. More women than men attended. Oliver wanted it that way. He had no desire to compete with other men for the best-looking women.

By 11:00 p.m., the Conrad mansion was overflowing with alcohol, food, music, conversation, and what many had come for - sex. Oliver always hired a six-piece band to set up and play in the back parlor for guests who wanted to dance. He spared no expense. He made sure his guests had a good time. Conversation usually centered on what was going on in current events. Tonight it was discussions about Jackie Robinson, the first African-American professional baseball player, The Truman Doctrine, and the first plane to break the sound barrier.

Eli Conrad was a frugal man. Air conditioning exceeded his budget. Only room air conditioners existed in the second-floor bedrooms. The main floor used ceiling fans to cool each room. On warm summer nights, the living areas and kitchen were stuffy and uncomfortable. Oliver's parties, which now attracted 50 to 60 people, taxed the house's ability to be cooled. It wasn't unusual to find half of the guests on the front porch or in the back yard. Tables and chairs were set up to handle those who chose to leave the house.

"Al - glad you could come tonight," Oliver said, as he shook Al Savuzzo's hand.

"Wouldn't miss one of your parties for the world, Oliver."

"Hey, thanks for the tip on the property in Downer's Grove. I think it's going to be a gold mine."

Savuzzo had information about the foreclosure on a piece of

commercial real estate that could be turned in a matter of weeks. It would make Oliver a substantial amount of money.

"Remember our deal," Al replied.

"I know. You get 25% of the profit. I take the risk."

"You got it. Glad to see you're so timely with your monthly payments," Al added. "Now, where's the bar?"

Al knew where the bar was. He'd been to numerous Conrad parties. He looked forward to Saturday night all week. Nothing would keep him from one of Oliver's parties.

"I love that "39 Caddy. Aren't you glad it wasn't in the driveway when we torched your car?" Al laughed.

"Ah, yeah, that car is one of a kind," Oliver replied.

It wasn't long before Oliver picked out someone to focus his attention on. Molly Simmons was the daughter of a wealthy Chicago attorney. Only 23 years old, she looked older than her age. Her short blond hair and fair complexion caught his attention. He watched her as she ordered a drink from the bar. Her dress fit tightly to her well-proportioned body.

"Hi, my name's Oliver - you are?"

"Molly, Molly Simmons."

"I'm your host. I just wanted to welcome you."

"Thank you. Is this your home?"

"Yes, it is. Do you like it?"

"It's beautiful," Molly responded.

"Would you like a tour?"

"Yes, thanks."

Oliver spent the next hour giving Molly a tour of the Conrad mansion. It wasn't the first time he'd picked out a young, attractive woman. It was his usual approach. The rest of the night, they were inseparable. Whether it was dancing in the parlor or sharing drinks on the porch, they were always together. Oliver was good at wooing women. He didn't want a relationship, just one night of pleasure. What he hadn't expected was the appearance of Molly's sister. Arriving late due to another engagement, she found them cuddled on a couch on the third floor.

"Molly, I need to get you home. Let's go," Susan Simmons said.

Susan was a beautiful woman in her own right. She had attended one of Oliver's earlier parties and knew what they were about. When word leaked to her that her younger sister would be attending, she decided to show up.

"Susan this is Oliver - he's the host."

"I know Oliver. I came to one of his parties last month. Why do you think I'm here?"

Oliver sat silently watching the sisters. He knew his evening was over. Within minutes, Susan escorted Molly from the grounds.

"Hey, Oliver, looks like you bombed tonight," Al said as he watched Molly leave.

"Yep. Not so good tonight, but the night's still young."

It was 1:00 a.m. Oliver had failed to connect with Molly Simmons.

"Laynie, I'm going out to take the Caddy for a ride. I'll be back in 30 minutes."

"You okay to drive?" Laynie asked.

"Yeah, I'm fine."

Laynie had spent the night picking up after people. The job was endless. As soon as she felt like she'd caught up, she'd find more trash. Most in attendance never noticed her. Al Savuzzo did. He'd been to several of Oliver's parties and had always admired Laynie's looks. Even though she purposefully dressed conservatively, he could tell she hid a beautiful body underneath her cleaning smock. When Oliver left, Al decided to engage Laynie in conversation.

"Laynie - rough night tonight?"

"I'm used to it," she replied.

"Well, you do a great job."

"Thank you, Mr. Savuzzo."

"Call me Al."

"Sure - thank you, Al."

Laynie finished picking up and headed to the kitchen to start doing dishes. Al followed.

"Mind if I join you?"

"Mr. Savuzzo - I mean Al - you don't need to help. I'll be fine," Laynie responded.

"Nonsense, I insist."

Al was married with two children. In his mind, he was happily married, but there was something about Laynie Jessup. An exotic beauty, she attracted admiring stares from virtually every man who attended a Conrad party. Only Al had the nerve to act on it.

Chapter Twenty-One

Oliver rode around the neighborhood for nearly an hour. He needed to burn off the frustration of being jilted by Molly, thanks to Susan. When he returned, he decided to park the car in the garage. On his way out, he pulled down the garage door. He rejoined the party and planned to cover the car with the tarp the next morning. As he entered the kitchen, Laynie, with assistance from Al, was carrying trash out to dump behind the garage.

"Is he behaving?" Oliver asked.

"So far," she replied.

Al had been a perfect gentleman. From the time Oliver left, he had been helping Laynie clean up. Now he was hauling trash out to the trashcans in the alley.

"Let me carry that," Al said to her, as he took one of the bags from her shoulder.

Oliver walked into the den, sat in the chair across from the fireplace, and poured himself a glass of brandy. Within minutes, the brandy began working. Soon, he was asleep. No one paid any attention to him. Most of the guests had cleared out by 2:30 a.m. Al left at 2:00 a.m. When he woke up, Laynie was gone. He hadn't seen her since returning from his ride. When the last guest left, he started to go from room to room, searching for her. His final stop was the garage. He needed to place the tarp back on the Caddy. Pulling up the garage door he saw nothing unusual until he reached the back seat of the car. Lying on her side in the back seat was Laynie. Oliver got in next to her and gently tapped her on the shoulder.

"Laynie, it's Oliver. What happened?"

She opened her eyes but looked away.

"I'm okay. I was tired, and it was noisy inside, so I decided to lie down in the car. I hope that's okay. I didn't hurt the car."

"Laynie, don't worry about it. You can nap in this car anytime you want."

Oliver put his head back and closed his eyes. Soon, he was asleep.

It was 7:30 a.m. when he woke up.

"Laynie, Laynie," he called out.

She was gone. He got out of the car and went into the house. It was Sunday morning, and the house was spotless. A note awaited him on the kitchen counter.

Oliver, I'm sorry. Thank you for being there for me last night. I've gone to church. Will be back in a while. Laynie

She'd gotten out of the car sometime during the night and cleaned the house. Oliver shook his head.

Laynie went to church every Sunday. She made her life about her work and her church. They gave her comfort and occupied her mind. When she returned home from church, she prepared one of Oliver's favorite meals - pot roast, new potatoes, and green beans.

"Laynie, you didn't have to make dinner," Oliver said, as he walked into the kitchen.

"I know. I just wanted to," she replied.

"Can we eat in here?"

"Sure, as long as you don't make a mess," she laughed.

"If I do, I'll clean it up," he replied.

"That's a deal," she said, shaking her head.

Dinner was comfortable. They talked about Laynie's church and the impact it had on her life.

Oliver was starting to have feelings for her. He started to imagine what it would be like to be with her. He was drawn to her. He knew it couldn't work, but he couldn't help himself. He didn't know how Laynie felt about him, but he had a feeling she felt the same.

"Let's grill out tomorrow night. I have the day off. It'll just be you and me. What do you say?" Oliver asked.

The invitation shocked her. She'd known Oliver for years. She wanted there to be more between them. It just never felt realistic. Something had happened. She didn't know what, but she liked where it seemed to be going.

"Okay, that sounds nice," Laynie replied.

"Good. I'll get a good bottle of wine. We can sit out on the front porch after dinner."

"But what about your party?" Laynie asked.

"No more parties," Oliver replied. "It's time to end that phase of my life."

Laynie smiled as she washed the dishes. It was what she had hoped for several years. It had been hard watching Oliver with other women.

"Can I dry?" Oliver asked.

"Sure, if you want to."

Chapter Twenty-Two

The next night couldn't come quickly enough for Oliver. He purchased two steaks and two good bottles of red wine. It had been a long time since he'd been so nervous. He wanted the night to go well. During the day, he occupied himself by working at the hospital, finishing notes on cases he'd completed the previous week. He didn't want to spoil the special nature of the evening by being around too much during the day. As he walked down the steps to the kitchen, his hands shook. Laynie was preparing new potatoes when he walked in. It wasn't the same Laynie that he'd become accustomed to. In the place of a kitchen smock, she wore a light yellow sundress exposing a hint of cleavage. Her hair was down. It flowed over her shoulders. He'd never seen her with her hair down. He hesitated when she asked him to start the charcoal.

"Ah, sure - I'll do it right now," he said nervously.

Walking out the back door, he stumbled over the stoop. Laynie smiled. She knew he was nervous.

"You okay?" she asked.

"Yeah, I'm just clumsy."

"The steaks are in the refrigerator. I put some seasoning on them. I hope you'll like them."

"I'm sure I will," he answered.

Oliver didn't want to look uncomfortable. He wanted to impress her. Thus far, he thought to himself, he hadn't. Purposely, he stayed outside while he grilled the steaks. He didn't want to do anything else that would show how nervous he was. He needed the time to gather himself.

"Steaks ready?" Laynie asked as she came out on the back porch.

"Five minutes, and we'll be ready," Oliver replied. "Medium well, right?"

"Yes, how did you know?"

"Hey, give me credit. I pay attention."

Laynie smiled a warm, affectionate smile.

"Steaks are ready," Oliver said, as he walked into the kitchen five minutes later.

Laynie was in the dining room. She'd set the table and placed the remainder of the meal in the center. Oliver's place was set at the head of the table and Laynie's next to him.

"Wow, this really looks nice."

"I just thought it would be nice to fancy it up a bit. Is that okay?" she replied.

"Absolutely."

For the next hour, they enjoyed each other's company. The conversation was light and uncomplicated. Laughter was abundant. Each felt a particular closeness to the other. Race never mattered. Oliver saw Laynie as a beautiful, intelligent, active, loving woman whom he was fortunate to know. Laynie, for her part, saw Oliver as a caring, warm, sensitive, protective, handsome man who had become important to her.

"Let's go out on the front porch," Oliver suggested.

"Okay - should I get some wine glasses?"

"Yes, and I'll get the wine."

Oliver pulled the two Adirondack chairs together. He opened the wine and poured. Sitting back in the chairs, they toasted.

"To a better future," Oliver said.

"To a past that brought me to this house," Laynie replied.

"Laynie, you've never talked about your past. What brought you to us?"

"Well, let's see, I was 16 when I answered your father's ad. I moved here from Macon, Georgia. I'm one of 12 children. My father died when I was six. My mother didn't have enough to feed us all. She worked three jobs, but it wasn't enough. I left to make it easier for her and to be able to send money back home."

"I'm ashamed that I never asked. Can you forgive me?"

"Of course; it's not a big deal. It's just who I am," Laynie replied.

"Do you still send money home?"

"Yes, every week. I haven't heard from my mother in a couple weeks, but I send it no matter what."

Oliver shook his head.

"Are you okay?" Laynie asked.

"Yes, I'm just scolding myself."

"Why?"

"Because I should have known this."

Laynie laughed. She knew Oliver's intent was pure. He need not have apologized, but it was sweet. As she sipped her wine, she thought to herself that it was for the best. Lying to Oliver would protect him if something happened. Laynie Jessup wasn't from Macon, Georgia, but rather Mobile, Alabama. The story she told about her mother and family was true. What she said about her father wasn't. He was alive and living in Mobile. For the year prior to her leaving, he sexually molested her on several occasions. She didn't want Oliver to know the truth. It was too embarrassing.

"Do you hear from your siblings?" he asked.

"Not much. They have their own lives."

"How long has it been since you saw your mother?"

"Let's see, I guess eight years ago. You were away at college. I went to Macon to see her. Your father gave me a few days off. She thanked me for the money I sent. That was the last time."

"Did you like my father?" Oliver asked.

"Your father gave me a chance at a new life. He was tough. I know, because I watched him discipline you, but he loved you. Don't ever think he didn't."

"I never saw that. He was distant, aloof, and hardly ever there," Oliver commented.

"He had to fight every day of his life. He wanted a good life for you.

Don't judge him too harshly."

Oliver sat quietly, thinking about Eli. He hardly knew his father.

"Look, a firefly," Laynie pointed out.

"Yeah, I see it," Oliver replied.

"We used to sit on the back porch and try and count them. My brothers would poke holes in Mason jar tops and catch them. You get six or seven in a jar, and it's like having a flashlight."

"Mason jars? You caught fireflies in Mason jars in Macon, Georgia?"

"Ha ha, funny man," Laynie laughed.

"Okay don't hate me, but I used to catch them and pull their tails off," Oliver replied.

"That's awful! Why?"

"I used to pinch off the blinking part to make a ring. It would stick on my finger due to the gooey stuff inside. It made a cool, blinking ring."

"Oh, my God - you have to be kidding. That's gross," Laynie replied, looking away.

"I know, but I was a lonely child in a strict home. What did you expect?"

Laynie started to laugh. She hadn't felt this good in a long time.

"Oliver, you're so full of it."

"Yeah, I know. What can I say?"

For the next three hours, they sat talking, laughing, and drinking wine. It was past midnight. The sky was clear, and the stars were bright.

"Damn, that's a bright sky," Oliver commented.

"I know. Makes me feel really small," Laynie said, as she looked up at the sky.

"What do you mean?"

"I don't know. It seems like we're just here for a blink of the eye in comparison to the universe and everything around us," Laynie remarked.

"Wow, that's deep," Oliver said, as he poured her another glass of wine.

"I know. I tend to get a bit philosophical. Sorry."

"No, that's great. You're like me. I do that all the time."

"Do you ever think about why you're here?" Laynie asked.

"Yes, but I just count on there being a plan," Oliver answered. "Hey, I think I've kept you up long enough. Tomorrow's Sunday, and I know you'll be going to church."

"I feel bad that you cancelled your party."

"Are you kidding? You're looking at a different person. This is way better than any party."

Laynie didn't want the night to end. Neither did Oliver.

"Let me walk you to your room," Oliver said, as he helped her to her feet.

"Okay, but what about the dishes?"

"They'll wait till tomorrow. I'll take care of them. Don't worry."

Standing in front of Laynie's bedroom, Oliver had an overwhelming desire to kiss her. *Too soon*, he thought to himself, as he turned to leave. Laynie reached out for him. He turned, and she pulled him toward her. The embrace was warm, soft, and sensual. Laynie wanted him. She had for a long time. Their first kiss was beyond anything Oliver could have imagined. Her lips were soft and moist. Laynie reached for Oliver's hand and led him into her bedroom.

"Are you sure?" Oliver asked.

She didn't respond. Laynie placed her finger to Oliver's lips as if to say, "hush". She kissed him again and guided him to her bed. Their lovemaking was gentle, slow, and affectionate. Oliver had never experienced anything like it.

Chapter Twenty-Three

Present Day

James Conrad opened the first of three boxes full of pictures that had been stored in the basement of his father's home. It was difficult carrying on a normal conversation with Victoria ever since returning from Oliver's. He struggled to think of things to talk about. She could tell something was on his mind.

"Sweetheart, would you mind if I do some work in the den tonight?" James asked.

"No, I'll go upstairs and watch television in our bedroom."

Sitting at his desk, he pulled out a handful of pictures. They brought back memories of his youth as he thumbed through them. Only a few puzzled him. When he came upon the two that included Anthony Savuzzo, he removed them and placed them in the top drawer of his desk. Jason's earlier questions about the pictures had made him uncomfortable. He decided to keep them under lock and key. His primary focus was looking for pictures of Oliver and Miriam and anyone around them. After looking at all the pictures, he pulled out a dozen that he wanted to examine further.

Two of the pictures, clearly older than the others, were of Oliver as a teenager. Both were taken in front of the Conrad mansion. Each picture showed a housekeeper in the background. Under a magnifying glass, James could tell it was an African-American female. He searched his memory but couldn't remember his parents having servants. He remembered a conversation that he'd had with his father several years before he died.

"Dad, why didn't you have servants?" James had asked. "You could afford them, yet, except for Frederick, your driver, I don't ever remember us having a servant."

"That's right, I didn't need one. Neither did Miriam when she was alive," he replied. "James, you don't have any. I could ask you the same question."

"True - we just want to do the work ourselves. Guess we're like you."

"Don't you mean *Victoria* likes doing the work herself?" Oliver asked, chuckling.

"Yes, she insists on doing things herself. Did you *ever* have servants?"

"Once, but it didn't end well. I prefer not talking about it," Oliver responded.

James knew his father. When he said he didn't want to talk about it, he meant it. The conversation was over. The subject never came up again.

The servant in the picture had to be the one he referred to, James thought to himself. From the year printed on the back of the picture, it was clear that it had been taken 11 years before Oliver met and married Miriam. James concluded that whatever happened that changed Oliver's attitude about having servants must have taken place during that 11 year period.

"What happened? What went wrong to make it end badly?" James said aloud to himself.

Reaching into his desk, he pulled out the pictures that included Anthony Savuzzo. Anthony, the youngest of Al Savuzzo's children, had been James's best friend in college. As fraternity brothers, they had formed their own group of friends. Anthony was the leader. Oliver hadn't approved of the friendship and tried to dissuade any contact. James disobeyed. Anthony, better known as Tony Z to his friends, had an uncanny ability to draw people to him. Few who entered his circle and were accepted ever left. They were good days, James thought - days when the only thing they worried about was picking up girls and passing pop quizzes. James had always felt like Tony had sought him out. It was as if he'd been searching for him.

Returning his attention to the pile of pictures, he pulled out the two with the servant. He wanted to know more. He put them in a file and decided to share them with Jason and Claire in the morning. He sat alone trying to recall anything that would help identify the baby or what might have happened. All he knew for sure was that, according to the newspaper that was found in the trunk, it happened on or after March 18th, 1948. He knew that his parents had married in 1949 and that, a year later, he was born.

"I know my parents. There isn't any way that this happened after they were married. It had to happen between 1947 and 1948," he mumbled.

James and Claire arrived early. Each was anxious to see what the others had come up with. Jason was sitting on the front porch when they arrived.

"Before we sit down, I want to show you something," Jason said.

Leading them back to the garage he opened the garage door.

"Wow - still looks great," James remarked, looking at Oliver's Cadillac.

"I didn't know Grandfather had this," Claire stated.

"Oh, yeah. This was Oliver's baby. He bought it back in the mid-'40s. It was one of only a few that GM produced to celebrate their Golden Anniversary," James replied.

"Did you ever get to drive it?" Jason asked.

"No, he wouldn't let me touch it," James answered. "In fact, he forbade me from coming in here. It was like there was something evil in this garage."

"What do you mean?" Claire asked.

"I remember, when I was a little boy, he'd invite me to come watch him tinker with the Caddy, but, when I got to be about five, he changed. It was like it was a bad memory that he just couldn't get past. I don't know why, but he lost interest."

"Claire, can you help me pull up the tarp?" Jason asked.

"Sure."

Walking back to the house, James turned and looked at the garage and wondered what had made his father lose interest in his greatest pleasure.

James had brought all the pictures with him, except two. They sat down in the dining room and spread them out. He pointed out the two that contained the image of the servant.

"Do you know who that is?" Jason asked.

"Haven't the foggiest. I asked Dad about servants. All he would say is he had one once, but that it had gone badly."

"Granddad had a servant? He was always so against having servants. I figured that was why you and Mom were against it," Claire commented.

Jason looked at the picture.

"Wow, she was beautiful."

"Let me see," Claire said as she took the picture from Jason's hand. "You're right, she was."

"What we have to do is figure out who could possibly have had access to this house during the mid-'40s," James pointed out.

"Wait a minute. We don't know it was the mid-'40s. Just because the newspaper was there isn't proof. Someone could have placed it there to throw anyone off who found it," Jason remarked.

"I disagree," Claire responded. "The trunk was like a coffin. Did you see the baby clothes, toys, and blankets, how they were arranged? Whoever did this, did it with care. The paper was like a headstone."

"Good point," Jason replied.

"Jason, can you try to access employment records to see if you can identify this person?" James asked, pointing to the photo.

"Okay; it'll probably be tomorrow, since all government offices are closed."

"What do you want me to do, Dad?" Claire asked.

"Go check on Jackson - see how his work is coming?"

"What are you going to do?" Claire asked.

James knew who he needed to speak to. It wasn't something he wanted to do. He couldn't be honest with his children. Too much was at stake. He needed to visit with Alphonse Savuzzo. Anthony's father was still alive. At 93 years of age, he was in failing health. He hadn't left the Savuzzo compound in more than 10 years.

"I'm going to track down Frederick. Maybe he knows something," James answered.

"Where is Frederick?" Jason asked.

"Well, he left after Dad died. I don't know if he's still alive. I'm going to try to find him."

"Good idea," Claire responded.

Chapter Twenty-Four

It was past noon when James and Claire left. Jason picked up the flowers he'd purchased the day before for Alyssa's grave and headed to the cemetery. On his way, he tried to clear his head. His new relationship with Halie and the mystery of the discovery in the trunk had been constantly on his mind. As he settled into his lawn chair, he heard footsteps approaching.

"Mind if I pull up a chair?" Dan asked.

"Of course not. Beautiful Sunday, isn't it?"

"That it is," Dan nodded in agreement.

Dan unfolded his lawn chair and sat down next to Jason.

"Beer?"

"You brought a cooler to the cemetery?"

Dan hesitated.

"Sure, why not?"

Jason chuckled. He and Dan had gotten close over the past three years.

"Have your talk with Alyssa yet?"

"Not yet - just getting comfortable," Jason replied. "So, what do you have to tell her today?"

"Today, I'm here to tell her I'm in love. I wanted to thank her for setting me up with Jane."

"That's really great, Dan. So, when do you go to Wilmington?"

"I leave tomorrow."

Dan was in love. He and Jane had communicated every day since she'd returned home. It wasn't something that he planned or expected. Every day when he woke, he looked forward to hearing from her. Her voice made him feel better. She made him feel like the best might yet be ahead. They talked about long-distance relationships when she visited Chicago. Neither wanted to voice the genuine concern they both had about whether it could work. For now, they were happy seeing each other every couple of weeks.

"Okay, I'll start," Dan said.

"Alyssa, it's Dad. Hold on to your socks, but you did it. One of your fix-ups actually worked. I'm in love," Dan said, directing his conversation toward Alyssa's gravestone.

Jason listened. He knew Alyssa would be pleased to know her father had found someone. He hated not being able to confide in him about the discovery of the remains. For the next 30 minutes Dan told her about Jane, the week they spent together, plans for his visit to North Carolina, and his concerns about a long-distance relationship.

"So what do you think Alyssa would want you to do?" Jason asked.

"Knowing Alyssa, she'd tell me to move to Wilmington. I can hear her voice now. *Dad, do you love her? If so, everything else is unimportant. Go to her. Move!"*

"Why don't you?"

"Ah, because I'm a big city cop with a *wet behind the ears* detective that I constantly have to watch out for."

"Wet behind the ears? Did you say *wet behind the ears?"* Jason laughed.

"Oh yeah. You have a lot to learn yet. Don't get too cocky."

They both laughed.

"Okay, your turn," Dan said, looking at Jason.

Jason had much to tell but hesitated to open up for fear that Dan would pick up on his demeanor. He decided to stick to his new and growing relationship with Halie.

"Hey, Alyssa. I miss you babe. I love you. I don't know where to start."

Dan felt a tear building up. He knew how difficult the conversation would be.

"I've fallen in love. Guess your dad and I are a lot alike. Our timing's been eerily close," Jason said. "Let me tell you about her. I know I gave you a little bit of information when we first dated, but you deserve to know everything."

"No new news besides Halie?" Dan asked, as Jason finished.

"No," Jason replied. "Hand me a beer."

Dan knew his son-in-law. He knew something was on his mind and that he was holding back.

"You okay?"

"Yeah, I'm fine - just a little distracted."

"Anything I can do?"

"No, not right now, but if there is, I'll come to you," Jason replied.

The two sat in their chairs and spent the next hour talking about everything from the Chicago Cubs baseball team to proposed healthcare changes. It was relaxing, especially with Alyssa there.

"Okay, I'm out of beer, so we'd better wrap this up," Dan remarked.

"Yeah, I need to get going, too," Jason replied. "When do you leave tomorrow?"

"About 8:00 a.m. I get to Wilmington at 2:00 p.m. Be back in a week."

"Are you going to see Melinda and Kenny?"

"We're having dinner with them on Tuesday. Jane also wants to have dinner with Linda Phister. They're pretty close."

"Brings back memories," Jason remarked.

"I know. I think I'll go see Jasper Ogden while I'm there. Kenny said he's doing well since he came back to UA," Dan remarked.

"Kenny - hell I'm surprised he keeps up with anything at UA," Jason commented.

"I'll tell you what - if you need information, Kenny's the man to go to," Dan responded.

Jason sat up in his chair. *Why hadn't I thought of it sooner?* he thought to himself. Kenny could find out who the servant in the picture was. If he couldn't, nobody could.

"Hey Dan, have a great time in North Carolina, and, please, use protection," Jason laughed.

Dan shook his head. He was used to Jason's sense of humor. He gave it back to him when he could.

On his drive back home, Jason placed a phone call.

"Kenny, it's Jason."

"Jason Conrad - I'll be damned. How are you, buddy?"

"Who is it?" Melinda could be heard in the background

"Tell her it's the IRS. We're auditing her father and need her help."

Kenny laughed and handed the phone to Melinda.

"That you, Jason? How are you?"

"I'm great, Melinda. How are you guys doing?"

"We're the same. Study, study, study," she answered.

"Ouch - I don't miss that a bit," Jason replied

"Hey, any new women in your life?"

"Okay, how'd you know?" Jason asked.

"A little bird," Melinda answered.

"That little bird's name happen to be Jane Moran?"

"You got me. Dan told her. She told us."

Jason knew it would be hard to keep secret, especially with Dan now dating Jane. He didn't care.

"Her name's Halie. She's a school teacher."

"Tell me more," Melinda demanded.

"Well, she's beautiful, nice, intelligent, warm, caring, etc, etc, etc," Jason responded.

"Sounds like you might be in love."

"I am. I won't deny it."

"I'm glad for you," Melinda said warmly.

"Thanks. Can I talk to Kenny for a minute?"

"Yes, but first tell me you'll help us get residencies in Chicago."

"Consider it done. Let me know what you're looking for. I'll pull my extensive strings," Jason laughed.

Jason did have powerful influence in the Chicago medical community. Not because of him but, rather, his family.

"Jason, what do you need?"

"Your IT talents, Kenny."

"How can I help?"

"I need you to hack into the employment records for Hinsdale, Illinois, or perhaps Chicago or Cook County. I need to find someone. They worked for my grandfather Oliver in the early to mid-'40s. Can you do that?" Jason asked.

"I'll give it my best shot," Kenny replied. "Do you have a name?"

"No - all I know is she was a servant in the house. I think she was the only female servant Oliver had."

"Wow; this will be tough, but I'll try."

"Knowing you, that's plenty good enough," Jason responded. "Hey, I hear you're having dinner with Dan Tuesday night."

"Yeah, he called last week."

"Do me a favor. Don't mention any of this to him. It's a family thing. Can you do that?" Jason asked.

"Sure - no problem."

Chapter Twenty-Five

Dan Johnson looked forward to his trip to Wilmington. It was a late July day, and the temperature had already hit 80 degrees by 7:30 a.m. As he waited for his flight he thought about how much his life had changed. The tragedy of his daughter's death had brought him together with Jane. It was an odd twist of fate – but one that Alyssa would have believed possible.

Waiting in airports for flights never bothered Dan. He loved watching people. Sitting quietly, he enjoyed imagining where his fellow passengers were headed. *So many people,* he thought to himself, *each with their own story*. In the seat to his right sat a young mother with two small children. Standing against the wall, a middle-aged man read a newspaper. Across from him, an elderly couple sipped Starbuck's coffee. No one sat next to each other. Everyone left the seat beside them empty. It was as if no one wanted anyone too close. Some people went as far as to place luggage beside them to dissuade anyone from attempting to sit down. Only when the room filled did people open up the seats next to them.

"Wow - it's just like being in an elevator. Nobody talks. Everyone's afraid to speak to the person next to them," Dan said aloud to himself.

"Did you say something?" the woman two seats away asked.

"No, I'm sorry; I was just talking to myself."

"Well, tell yourself you're right. It's not as friendly a world as it once seemed," she responded. "Although, I can't say it ever was."

"Good point," Dan replied.

Dan was seated in a window seat in the back of the plane. He planned to sleep the first leg and look at case materials he brought on the second. As the plane leveled off, he closed his eyes and leaned against the window. The passenger next to him awakened him.

"Sir, are you okay?"

"I'm fine - why?"

"You were having a nightmare. You were flailing away pretty good there," the middle-aged businessman said to him.

He'd dreamed about seeing Alyssa on the gurney the day she died. He could see her innocent face as they pulled the sheet back up to cover her for the ride to the morgue. He twisted and turned in his seat trying to get away from the patrolman and reach out for his daughter.

"I'm sorry. I *was* having a nightmare. Hope I didn't hit you or anything."

"No, I was just worried you'd hurt yourself."

Dan decided he'd best stay awake the rest of the trip.

Jane was waiting for him in the baggage area. As he came off the escalator she walked up to him and put her arms around him.

"Wow, I really needed that."

"Rough flight?" Jane asked.

"Bad nightmare. Guy next to me had to wake me up so I wouldn't punch anyone out."

"I'm sorry. What was it about?"

"Ah, the day we found Alyssa. It was complicated. I'm glad he woke me up."

"Well, let's focus on having a good time, okay?" Jane said.

"I'm counting on it."

Dan loaded his suitcase into the trunk of Jane's car and headed to her house.

"So, what are the plans this week? You've got me all week," he laughed.

"I'm glad. I took a week's vacation. I thought we'd spend some time on the beach, have dinner with friends here in Wilmington, and just relax and enjoy each other."

"That sounds great to me," Dan replied.

After emptying his suitcase, Dan met Jane on the back porch.

"You know, I think it's cooler today in North Carolina than it's supposed to be in Chicago. I think we're going to hit the upper 90s," Dan remarked.

"See all the advantages of living in the south?" Jane laughed, as she handed him a beer.

"Yeah, I know," Dan chuckled.

"So, bring me up to date. What's going on in your life? Tell me about Jason's new girlfriend."

Dan knew the questions would come.

"Hey, you spilled the beans to Melinda and Kenny. Jason told me they already knew. He thinks I told you," Dan related.

"Ah, you did tell me, and you never said it was a secret."

Dan paused.

"Oh yeah, you're right."

Jane knew most of what was going on. Dan had read Jason's face when he talked to Alyssa at the cemetery. He knew he'd slept with Halie.

"Well, there really isn't much to tell. I do believe Jason and Halie have been together, if that's what you want to know," he asked.

"That and much more," Jane replied. "Is he happy?"

"Yes, very much so. I'm glad to say."

Jane smiled. She'd watched the agony that both of them had suffered when Alyssa died.

"You and Jason went through a lot, Dan. I'm glad you have each other and that you've found people who love you."

Dan leaned over and kissed her. They spent the rest of the afternoon enjoying each other. The absence had heightened the desire. When they woke from a nap, it was 9:00 p.m.

"Oh wow - I think we were a bit tired," Jane said.

"Jane, what we did made us tired, and it was a good tired."

Jane laughed and pulled the sheet up.

"I don't think we're done yet," she chuckled.

Dan's phone started to beep as he began kissing her.

"Sorry, I have to get that. The cop in me."

"Dan, this is Herman Wise. You in Wilmington?"

"Hey, Herman, yes - I got in this afternoon."

"You staying with Jane?" Herman asked.

"Wow - this *is* a small town," Dan replied. "Yes, I'm staying with Jane."

"We going to have lunch tomorrow?"

"I'm looking forward to it," Dan answered. "Tarheels" at noon, right?"

"Yep, see you there."

Jane and Dan continued what they had started and never made it out of bed till the next morning. It was 8:00 a.m. when Jason finally contacted them.

"Hey, Dan. Where you been? Haven't heard from you."

"It's only been a day. Can't you get by a day without me there?" Dan asked.

"Oh, we try. It's really hard. All the guys keep asking where their good buddy is," Jason kidded.

"Well, you know, I think you'll just have to step into my shoes. I think I'm going to take a job as a County Sheriff down here."

Jane heard it all. As soon as Jason hung up, she looked at Dan.

"That's not a bad idea, you know. You could learn to love the south."

"I'm sorry, Jane. I was just trying to get Jason to back off. I know we have to talk about the long-distance thing. Can we do it the day before I leave?"

"Sure - fine with me," Jane replied.

Both knew it was a huge issue. *Long distance rarely works,* Jane thought to herself. *Someone has to make the move if it's a good-enough relationship.* She knew what she had developed with Dan was. She just didn't know if she could bring herself to move.

Chapter Twenty-Six

Jason answered his phone on the first ring. It was Kenny.

"Hi, Kenny - what's up?"

"Jason, I need more information if you want me to find the person you're looking for."

"What do you need?"

"Well, give me the address where she lived. I also need any pertinent information about her. You know, where she worked, social security number - anything will help," Kenny replied.

"Okay, I'll work on it. I'll call you back by the end of the day. Hey, Kenny, I have one other person I'd like you to see if you can find. His name is Frederick Menick. He was Oliver's driver. He left after he died," Jason continued.

"Okay, I'll do my best."

"Where are you having dinner with Dan and Jane?" Jason asked.

"They're taking us to the Wilmington Grill. It's supposed to be one of Wilmington's best places."

It was 7:30 a.m. in Chicago. The heat had already started to build. Highs for the day were expected to be near 100. The drive into the 71st Precinct gave Jason time to think. He needed the information that Kenny was pursuing. His activities at that moment were outside the law. He had a duty to report what he'd found. His loyalty to his family overrode that duty.

Mixed in with his thoughts about the trunk were his new feelings for Halie. He had a new sense of contentment because of her. Nothing seemed so overwhelming knowing he would soon be with her. The pictures that they'd looked at together were now critical to discovering the truth. James had asked him to try to identify the servant from the photos. He intended to do that and more. If he could find Frederick Menick, he'd question him before James found him. One thing kept going through his mind. After looking at all the pictures in the boxes, he'd noticed that the two pictures of James with the unidentified young man were gone. He knew his father had lied about not knowing the man. There had to be a reason why he was covering up his identity. He was intent on finding the truth. He needed Dan's counsel.

Dan and Herman Wise had become friends.

"Herman, good to see you," Dan said as he joined Herman in a booth at Tarheels.

"Same here, Dan. How ya been?"

"Good - really good, in fact. But everybody in Wilmington knows that – right, Herman?"

"Well, if you're talking about Jane - yep, everybody knows. I will tell you we're all happy for you guys."

"Thanks, Herman. How's crime in Wilmington?"

"Been down ever since you left. I wonder why?" Herman laughed.

"I guess I just scared all the criminals away," Dan chuckled.

"Oh yeah - that's got to be it," Herman replied.

"All kidding aside, any word on Vince, Leon, and Anthony Savuzzo?"

"No, nothing new. Vince took a life-in-prison deal. Leon accidentally slipped on a shiv in the bathroom at the prison in Raleigh. Poor guy, kept falling on the same shiv, something like 12 times. Must of hit a bar of soap," Herman laughed.

"Leon's dead? I never heard that."

"Happened day before yesterday."

"Wow - guess it didn't work out too well for him," Dan replied.

Dan and Herman got caught up. As he listened, Dan tried to imagine working in a small town police department. He couldn't. The only solution was for Jane to move to Chicago.

"Kenny, you need to get ready. Dan and Jane will be here soon," Melinda called out.

"I will. Let me just finish one more thing."

Kenny was a master at a computer keyboard. Not much was out of his reach. Graduating number one in his medical school class was now a given. Students and faculty alike recognized his intelligence and good heart. It had taken Melinda two years to see Kenny's depth, but, once she did, she fell in love. Over the past two years, she'd spent far more time with Kenny's family than she had with her own. The desire to go on summer trips to Sweden with her parents was gone. She preferred spending her free time in Boone, North Carolina, with Kenny and the rest of the Conrow clan.

"Melinda, what do you think Jason's working on?"

"I don't know, why?"

"I have a funny feeling. Both the people he wants me to locate worked for his grandfather. I just wonder what's behind his interest in finding them."

"He must have a good reason," Melinda replied.

"I just hope he's not into something bad. He asked me not to mention what he wants to Dan."

"Not to Dan? Wow - that's a surprise. I thought he shared everything with Dan."

"I know. That's why I'm worried. He called me this afternoon and gave me more information about both people. He sounded different. I could tell he was working on something big," Kenny replied.

"Have you found anything yet?"

"I found Frederick Menick. He was easy. I found him through social security. He lives in Cicero, not far from Hinsdale, where Jason lives. I called Jason about an hour ago and told him. The housekeeper he wants me to find will be a lot harder. She was African-American, according to Jason. I don't think she ever registered with any governmental agency," Kenny related.

"Hmmm, I wonder how else you could find her?"

"You know, if it were Boone in the '40s, the one place African-Americans found peace was in their church," Kenny suggested.

"Call Jason - tell him that."

Kenny didn't wait long. He wasn't giving up. He was intent on finding the housekeeper through records, but he knew it might be faster to go the human route.

"Kenny, you forget something. I just talked to you," Jason said, as he answered his cell phone.

"I know. I was talking to Melinda, and we have an idea. I'm not saying I won't find the housekeeper, but it's going to be tough."

"What's your idea?"

"The place African-Americans went to in difficult times in the '40s and '50s was their church. Find out where the closest African-American church is to Hinsdale that operated in the fifties. Canvass them. See if anyone knows anything."

"Damn! That's a good idea, Kenny."

"If I were you, I'd get a local bus-route map and see if anything connected to Hinsdale. I doubt she drove. Most likely walked to a bus stop and took the bus to the nearest church."

"Okay, you're just too damn good at this, Kenny. Why don't you give up medicine and become a cop?" Jason asked.

"I would, but I don't think Melinda would be too crazy about it."

Jason hung up just as he pulled up in front of 1209 Grand Boulevard in Cicero, Illinois, Frederick Menick's home.

Chapter Twenty-Seven

Frederick Menick was 84 years old. He'd come to the United States in 1945 from Germany at the age of 18. As a youngster, he missed the frenzy of Nazi Germany. His home, Dresden, had been the target of an extensive British bombing raid. Thousands of lives had been lost and the city reduced to rubble. American Intelligence recruited his father, a scientist. He and his family had gotten priority relocation. Soon after arriving in the States, his father died of pneumonia. It was up to Frederick to support his mother and younger sister.

The Menick house was small and located in a rough neighborhood of Cicero. It was 6:00 p.m. and the heat of the day was at a peak. Temperatures hovered at 101 degrees and heat indexes hit 115. Jason, sitting in an air-conditioned car, was hesitant to get out. The house, tucked in between two eight-unit brick apartments, looked out of place. Jason opened his car door, looked around his surroundings, and began to walk up the front sidewalk. As he stepped up onto the porch, he noticed two lawn chairs. He searched for a doorbell and saw a hole in the white clapboard siding. Just as he was about to ring the bell, a tall, elderly man opened the door.

"May I help you?"

"Frederick, it's me, Jason Conrad. Remember, you picked Alyssa and me up at the airport four years ago. You helped us get the luggage to Oliver's guest quarters."

"Oh, yes. I remember you. It's been a while."

"May I come in? I have a couple questions I need to ask you."

"Sure."

Jason sat on the couch, Menick in a recliner that was clearly his favorite chair. The inside of the house smelled musty but appeared well kept. Everything seemed to have been recently cleaned. Jason could see into the kitchen, where dishes had been washed, dried, and neatly stacked.

"Frederick, whatever happened to your mother and sister?" Jason asked.

"My mother's dead. My sister moved to New York. She died of breast cancer."

"How long did you work for my grandfather?"

"Oh, my, let me think. I'd say it was in the mid to late '40s that I started there," he replied.

"You worked for him for more than 60 years. That's a long time."

"I know. Your grandfather was a good man - a tough man, but a good man."

"Do you ever remember any other servants working for him?"

Menick hesitated, appearing to be in thought.

"No, just me. He had a housekeeper once, but Miriam told me something happened, and she disappeared. They never hired another. I think the only reason your grandfather hired me was that he wanted someone around to make sure Miriam was safe."

Jason looked around the living room as Frederick spoke. Pictures sat in cabinets and stands. Some hung on the walls.

"Do you have any coffee, by chance?" Jason asked.

"Sure, it'll take a few minutes, but I can fix some for you, if you'd like."

Jason nodded his head in the affirmative, and Frederick moved into the kitchen. Jason wasn't interested in coffee. He just wanted a chance to look at the pictures. He had to do it quickly, before Menick returned.

"When was the last time you saw my father?" he called out as he inspected each picture.

"Oh, at the funeral," Frederick replied. "I think that's right."

Good, I made it here first, Jason thought to himself.

"You knew him pretty well, didn't you?" Jason asked.

"Not really, he was always on the go. He ran with a tight knit group."

Most of the pictures were of Frederick's mother, sister, and father. It appeared he'd never married and had very little contact with anyone. Walking back to his seat, Jason scanned a locked cabinet. One picture stood out - Menick standing next to Oliver and his red Cadillac with a figure in the background, the housekeeper.

"Hey, thanks for the coffee," Jason said, as Frederick rounded the corner with a tray.

"It was no problem."

"What was it like working for my grandfather all those years?"

"It was a pleasure. He and your grandmother were wonderful people. She was a real lady," he answered.

"And my grandfather?"

"A shrewd businessman – and a very tough person to get to know," Frederick replied.

"Did you ever meet anyone who seemed not to be legit?"

"You mean in a criminal way?"

"Yeah, I guess that's what I mean," Jason replied.

"No, never!"

"Did my grandfather or grandmother ever talk about any servants they used to have?"

"They didn't like having servants. I don't remember Miriam ever having someone to help her with the house."

"I really appreciate your spending some time with me, Frederick," Jason said as he got up to leave.

"I'm sorry about your wife."

"Thank you. It was a tough loss."

"I know. I've felt that before, too. You'll recover," Frederick responded.

The drive back to Hinsdale was second nature for Jason. It had to be, as his mind was focused on the photo in Menick's house. It clearly showed the housekeeper. Menick had lied. As he pulled away, his cell phone rang.

"Hey, Jason, it's Halie. How'd your day go?"

"Okay - busy, interesting. How was yours?

"Well, imagine 25 sixth-graders all trying to talk at once," Halie laughed.

"I have to tell you, I don't know how you do it. I think elementary teachers have the hardest jobs in the world. You know those polls that rank the toughest jobs? Commercial fisherman always ranks at the top. Trust me, they wouldn't last a day in a classroom," Jason admitted.

"Well, I'm glad you appreciate what I do," Halie responded. "Frankly, I think you have a really tough job."

"Yeah, well, I love it, as I know you love what you do."

"Hey, if you want to come over, I've got some pasta bolognese that I'm going to make. You can watch television while I grade papers."

"I'd love that. I'll stop at home and change and be over in 30 minutes."

"Perfect. I should have the pasta well on the way by the time you get here."

Jason needed to call his father. He decided to call him on the drive back to Hinsdale. There was no need for James to make the visit to Menick. He hoped he wouldn't be too upset that he hadn't been able to visit him first.

"Hey, Dad."

"Hi, Jason, what's up?

"Just wanted to let you know I just had a visit with Frederick Menick today."

"I thought that was my job," James remarked.

"Well, I got information about where he lives, so I just decided to save you the trouble."

"And did he say anything that helped?" James asked.

"Not really. He says he doesn't remember any servants working for Oliver. He said he felt like Oliver hired him only to protect Miriam."

"Hmm, guess that was a dead end," James replied.

James had wanted to see Menick first, but it wasn't crucial. He didn't think he had any information that would help. He had only mentioned his name to Jason to draw attention away from the person he really wanted to speak with - Al Savuzzo.

Chapter Twenty-Eight

Al Savuzzo's son Anthony had escaped unscathed from Leon Hingle's attempt to turn state's evidence. Vince had held firm. Anthony was safe to lead the Savuzzo family. His father, Al, was in ill health and unable. For more than 40 years, he'd led the family. Anthony now had taken his place. He was a highly intelligent, personable man who had a persuasive way about him. The same age as James Conrad, he had befriended him as a freshman at DePaul University. Throughout college, they were inseparable. Joining the Phi Theta Fraternity together was a given. The meeting and friendship weren't accidental. Al had directed his son to gain James's confidence and friendship.

Anthony was surprised when James called and asked for a meeting with his father.

"Tony, I'd like your permission to meet with Al. If you want to be there, it's fine, but I need to ask him some questions about my dad."

"What's this about, Jimmy?

"It's about something that happened before you and I were born."

"Tell me more," Anthony replied.

"I can't. I wish I could. It's really important."

"Okay, I'll set it up, but I want to be there."

James was pleased.

"Sure - when?"

"Come over this afternoon, say 3:00 p.m."

James sat at his desk and thought about the first time his friend had called and asked for help.

September 1977

Throughout medical school, James and Anthony had kept in touch on a weekly basis. Each still considered the other his best friend. Although they had pursued different careers, they'd stayed connected. Rumors had reached James about the Savuzzo family. It was hard to stay out of the limelight. Even so, James wasn't about to sever any relationship with his best friend. James had met and married Victoria. Anthony served as his best man. Oliver, having long since given up the effort to dissuade James from the friendship, grudgingly watched.

"James, you have a phone call. It's Tony," Victoria said.

Newly married, the young couple lived in an apartment on the north side of Hinsdale with their newborn son, William. James had taken a job with a small orthopedic group. He was beginning what would be a highly successful medical career.

"Jimmy, it's Tony. You have a minute?"

"Sure - what's up Tony?"

"I need your help."

"What do you need?" James asked.

"Can you meet me out front?"

"Okay. I'll head out now."

James hung up the phone and walked into the kitchen.

"Babe, I have to go out for a little while. Will you be okay here?"

"Sure. I'll be fine."

As he waited on the curb, he wondered what was wrong. He soon found out. Anthony pulled up in his 1977 Buick Riviera and stopped in front of the apartment.

"Get in," he directed.

James walked over, opened the door, and sat down.

"Damn, Tony - you're bleeding."

"Yeah, I know. I had a little accident. Can you help me?"

"We need to get you to a hospital."

Tony looked at James.

"No hospital. You can fix me up when I get home."

"I don't have any equipment," James replied.

"Then go back in the apartment, and get your medical bag."

Within minutes, James was back with his bag. Tony pulled away and reached the Savuzzo compound 10 minutes later. Bruno Caseo waved him in.

"Who's this?" Bruno asked.

"Jimmy Conrad," Tony replied, as the two men helped him into the house.

"You Doc's son?"

"If you mean Oliver, yes," James replied.

James knew who Bruno was.

"What happened?" Al Savuzzo asked.

"Ah, nothing; I tried to make a pickup and the guy went bonkers."

"What'd you do to him?"

"Nothing - he settled down and made the payment."

Anthony wasn't his father. He struck fear in those he dealt with, but he didn't resort to violence so easily. He preferred to try to reason with people. Most of the time, it worked. Sometimes it didn't. James inspected the wound. It was a slicing knife wound.

"You'll be fine, Tony. Probably take about 40 stitches, but it isn't so deep as to affect anything else," James remarked.

"Thanks, Jimmy; can you sew me up?"

"Sure. Let me numb it a bit. It's still going to hurt, so you might want a drink of scotch."

"You mean like we used to do at parties?"

"Yeah, but not for me, I'm doing the sewing."

James knew who Anthony was. More importantly, he knew he was his best friend. Anthony was someone he could always count on, no matter what. In turn, James would be that for Anthony. When Tony needed him, James knew he would be there.

Present Day

Walking up the stairs to Al's room, James had a feeling of gloom. He was afraid of what he might hear. It was now apparent that his father had been involved with Al. How, he didn't know. Tony stood at the top of the stairs.

"He's pretty aware right now. It's a good time to talk to him."

"Thanks, Tony."

James and Tony entered Al's room. He was awake and sitting up in bed. He'd rarely left the bed over the past six months. He knew his life would end soon. The good days were few and far between. The bad days were the norm.

"Hi, Mr. Savuzzo - how are you feeling today?" James asked.

Al looked at Tony, wondering who James was.

"Dad, you remember Jimmy Conrad, my best friend from college?" Tony asked.

"Oh, yeah, Oliver's kid," Al said, smiling.

"Right, Mr. Savuzzo. You knew my dad!"

"First, call me Al, and, yes, Oliver and I were friends. I used to go to his parties. They were a blast."

James was puzzled. He didn't know what the relationship between Al and his father had been.

"Al, I asked Tony if I could ask you a couple questions about my dad. Would that be okay?"

"Sure; what do you want to know?"

"Well, first, did you ever go to my dad's house in the mid '40s?"

"Are you deaf? I told you I went to his parties. He stopped them in the mid-'40s. Before that – wow! Oliver could throw a party. I met more women at his parties than anywhere."

James never knew the side of his father that Al was talking about.

This wasn't the father that he'd known. The man he knew was quiet, reserved, withdrawn, and a family man.

"When you attended Oliver's parties, did you ever see a servant or housekeeper?"

Al leaned back into his pillow. He looked out the window. He paused before saying anything.

"Housekeeper? No, I never knew Oliver to have a housekeeper."

"So you don't remember any servants?"

"Nope, except for the driver. I think his name was Frederick."

"You remember the driver?"

"Yeah, he was German, I think."

"What year was that?" James asked.

Al hesitated, searching his memory for the year.

"Probably 45' or 46' - I'm not sure."

"What did my father do for you?" James pressed.

"A little of this and a little of that," Al replied.

James hadn't expected Al to be forthright about his father's involvement.

"Jimmy, I think that's enough questions," Tony interrupted.

"Just a couple more, okay?"

"Okay, but just a couple."

"Al, did you ever see an African-American servant at Oliver's house?"

Al looked at Tony and then at James.

"No, never - I'm done. Leave me alone."

The question had struck a nerve. James knew it. So did Tony.

"Thank you, Mr. Savuzzo," James said, as he left the room.

"Yeah, get out," Al replied.

As they walked down the stairs, Tony turned to his good friend.

"What was that about?"

"Just an old family mystery that I thought your dad could help me solve."

"Why did you think my dad could help?"

"Tony - news flash. I've known about Oliver's involvement with your family for a long time. I just didn't know how he got involved. I have a pretty good idea now. Al's the only person old enough to have any knowledge of those days," James answered.

"Did your visit help?"

"Yes, more by what Al didn't say than by what he did. You saw it, Tony. He was hiding something," James commented. "I think he knew the housekeeper."

Chapter Twenty-Nine

July 1947

Laynie Jessup woke up in Oliver Conrad's arms. It was Sunday morning, and neither wanted to get out of bed. The night had been full of warmth and passion. More importantly, Laynie felt safe in his arms.

"Oliver, Oliver, are you awake?" Laynie asked.

"I am now," Oliver said, laughing.

"I need to get ready for church."

"Go ahead. Would you mind if I watched?"

"Sure - just stay in bed," Laynie replied.

As she moved over him to get up, she felt the warmth of his body touching her.

"I'm going to take a quick bath. Then I'll get dressed," she said.

"Can I join you?"

"No. Stay in bed. I'll be ready in a flash."

Oliver watched as she prepared her bath.

"Hey, are you asleep?" Laynie asked, as she tapped him on the shoulder.

Looking up, he realized that he'd fallen asleep. Laynie was dressed and ready to go to church.

"Damn, I'm sorry I drifted off," Oliver said, as he looked at her. "Wow! You're gorgeous."

"Hey, it's Sunday - watch your language. I'll see you after church, unless you'd like to go," Laynie said, as she kissed him goodbye.

"Maybe another Sunday - that okay?"

"Sure," Laynie replied.

Each Sunday, Laynie caught the 47 CTA Bus to Cicero. She'd found a church she liked that had become her spiritual home. It was only a 15-

minute walk to the bus stop, and she enjoyed the exercise and sunshine. As she walked toward the bus stop, Oliver lay in bed, thinking about his future. He stared at the ceiling. He felt a happiness that he hadn't experienced before.

"Wow, this feels so right. What have I been doing these last two years?" he said aloud to himself.

The last several days had changed him. Drifting back to sleep, his thoughts were of Laynie. He didn't notice when, two hours later, she crawled back into bed beside him. The smell of her hair awakened him, as he reached out to pull her into him. She smiled and kissed him gently on the cheek.

"Oliver, how can this work?"

"We can make this work. Don't worry - we can," he replied.

"Do you know all the barriers? People judge. They're cruel," she responded.

"Laynie, all I know is that I'm in love with you. I have been for a long time. I'm not about to let anything separate us."

With that he pulled her closer, holding her face in his hands.

"I love you, Laynie Jessup."

"I love you, too, Oliver."

Oliver was honest about his feelings and his intent. He committed himself to making their love last. Laynie, as she lay cupped in his arm, knew more than he that the odds were stacked against them. She knew he had no idea what he faced. Now their relationship was secret, *but what would happen in the light of day*? she thought to herself. She wondered if he could withstand the stares, whispers, and alienation he would face when they became public. Living life as an interracial couple in 1947 wasn't easy. Laynie had known several couples through her church. The judging came from both races. In 1947 it wasn't acceptable. It wasn't the norm. In addition, Oliver would have his profession to deal with. Physicians were expected to live according to societal standards. Veering away from those standards could mean the destruction of a career.

"Oliver, it's time to get up. It's past noon," Laynie said as she gently rubbed his arm.

"Past noon? I really did sleep well. I think having you next to me made the difference."

"Tell you what. You make the bed and get ready, and I'll cook breakfast. I brought in the Sunday paper. It's on the kitchen table."

As Oliver shaved and dressed, he made a decision. He wanted Laynie safe. With his schedule, he knew he'd be gone for periods of time. She would be alone. He decided to hire a driver, someone who could be there when he couldn't. Pulling up the sheets and arranging the pillows on Laynie's bed, he thought about the night he'd just experienced. He looked forward to a lifetime of nights in her arms.

"Hey, it smells great down here," Oliver said, as he entered the kitchen.

Laynie, serving the scrambled eggs, smiled.

"I hope you like it."

Dressed in a white cotton sundress, with her hair down over her shoulders, she looked like she belonged in Oliver's house. Her deep brown eyes showed emotion. Anyone looking at her knew what she was feeling. Oliver could see the happiness she felt at that moment.

"I made a decision upstairs. I hope it'll be okay with you, but I've decided to hire a driver."

"Why? We don't need one," Laynie responded.

"Well, I just don't like the idea of you being alone while I'm at work or when I'm called away. I'll feel much better about leaving if I know someone is here to help."

"You want them to live here?"

"Yes, I want you to move into my room and have them take the guest quarters," he replied.

"What will they do?"

"Anything you want, drive, help around the house, take care of the grounds. There's a lot to do around here."

"Oliver, I don't need the help. I'll be fine."

"I know you don't need the help, but do this for me, please?"

"Okay, just as long as they don't add more work for me," Laynie laughed.

Life for them settled into a routine over the next several weeks. It was a private life. Each hesitated to make their relationship public. Laynie had moved into Oliver's room. Days were filled with work. Nights became the time when they could be together. Eating in the kitchen, sitting on the front porch, looking at the stars, and making love drew them closer and closer.

Oliver advertised for a driver and set the date for the first interviews. He would conduct the interviews, but, at the end of each, he would introduce Laynie. He'd given a great deal of thought to the kind of person he wanted to hire. Not having built-in prejudices was the most important qualification. After interviewing seven candidates, he came to a realization. He needed to hire someone from outside the United States - someone not ingrained with racial bias and prejudice.

"Oliver, the next person's here," Laynie said as she stood at the entrance to the study.

"Okay, show him in."

Oliver stood and greeted the tall, young, blond man.

"Hello, my name is Oliver Conrad. Thanks for coming."

Nervous, the young man hesitated.

"Frederick Menick, Dr. Conrad. Pleased to meet you."

"Frederick, we call each other by our first names here. So, call me Oliver."

"Yes sir, Frederick replied.

"Tell me about yourself," Oliver asked.

"Well, I'm 20 years old. I came to the States from Germany two years ago. I live with my mother and sister. My father died a year after we got here," he answered.

"You left Germany after the second world war?"

"Yes, in 1945. I was 18 at the time," Frederick replied.

"That had to be hard."

"It was. We were lucky because my father was a scientist. The Americans made it easy to relocate."

"What did you think about what was going on in Germany before and during the war?" Oliver asked.

"My family hid our two Jewish neighbors for four years. Dresden was a beautiful, safe place until the bombing. We lost our home. My two older brothers died that night, as did our Jewish friends," Frederick explained.

"I'm sorry for your loss," Oliver responded.

"That's okay. It's been really hard on my mother. I think it killed my father's spirit. I'm ashamed of what Germany became. There were a lot of really good people who got lost and made bad decisions. We will never live it down."

"Why do you want this job?"

Frederick waited to answer, trying to formulate his words.

"I really need a job, sir, and a place to live. The ad you placed sounded like you were looking for someone who would do more than just drive. That's what I want. I want to stay busy and find a home."

"What have you been doing the past couple of years?"

"I've been working in the meat-packing district."

Oliver was familiar with the kind of work he was talking about. It was difficult, dangerous, and hard on a man's body and spirit. He understood how someone would want to get out and experience something different.

"Well then, you know what it's like to work hard," Oliver commented.

"Yes, sir, I do."

"When could you start?"

"Tomorrow, if you hire me," Frederick answered.

The final test was the most important. Oliver needed to see Frederick's reaction to a display of affection between Laynie and him. The look on his face and his reaction would tell him if he would be a good fit.

"Laynie, can you come in here for a second?" Oliver called out.

Laynie left the kitchen and walked into the den. Oliver reached for her hand. In a gentle, comfortable way, he pulled her into him and kissed her.

"Frederick, this is Laynie. She runs the place. She's the most important person in my life."

Oliver watched his reaction. He smiled as he surmised that Frederick was accepting and supportive. *He will do quite well,* he thought to himself.

"Hello, Ma'am - pleased to meet you."

"Call me Laynie."

"Laynie, Frederick starts tomorrow. Congratulations - you have the job," Oliver said, as he shook Frederick's hand.

Chapter Thirty

Present Day

Jason studied Halie's face as she graded papers. After interviewing Frederick Menick, he had stopped at his house only long enough to change clothes. He didn't want her to notice him looking at her for fear of making her feel uncomfortable. Her red hair, pulled back in a ponytail, was off her shoulders, exposing her neck. She wore no make-up. It was a casual evening, one that he'd enjoyed with Alyssa many times before. A small chicken-pox scar at the bridge of her nose was the only mark on Halie's face. Her complexion was smooth and unharmed by sun damage. Her mouth, in perfect balance with her face, was soft and sensual. Her eyes, bright green, caused people to stop when they saw her.

"Hey, are you checking me out?" Halie laughed, as she threw a pencil at him.

"I'm sorry, I was just looking at you. You're really beautiful."

"Yeah, sure - bet you noticed my chicken-pox mark, didn't you?" she asked.

"That's a character mark. Be proud of it."

Halie got up from the floor and moved over to the chair Jason was sitting in. She sat on his lap and put her arms around him.

"I'm so glad you're here."

"I'm glad you asked me to come by. It was an interesting day," Jason replied.

"What was interesting about it?"

"Oh, just a case I'm working on. Talked to an 80-year-old guy this afternoon. It was sad. He lives in this tiny house all by himself. He has to be lonely."

"My grandmother was like that. They learn to cope and to find things to occupy themselves," Halie responded.

"Still seems like an empty life. I'm glad I have you. I was like that man for the last three years."

"No, you weren't Jason. You suffered a great loss. It takes time. I'm just glad we met, because you've made me really happy. I get excited about each day, knowing there's a chance I may see you," Halie said, as she kissed him.

Jason held on to Halie tightly.

"Do you mind if I talk a little about Alyssa?" he asked.

"I'm glad you want to," Halie replied.

"The thing I regret the most is that I didn't listen. I was so consumed with my own life that I didn't pay attention to what was going on," Jason said. "If I had, I think she might still be alive. I'll never forgive myself for that."

"What do you think Alyssa would want? Do you think she'd want you to not forgive yourself? From everything I've heard, she was an amazing woman. She had the power to forgive and to love. You need to do that."

"How did I get so lucky?"

"I don't know. You probably owe Jeff a dinner," Halie replied.

"I wonder how Jeff and Kim are doing?" Jason pondered.

"Well, actually pretty good. I saw Kim at the mall a couple days ago. She told me they were living together."

"She actually moved in with him? He's a slob. I know him," Jason replied.

"Well, you have to admit he has a pretty cool place."

"Have you been there?"

"Do I hear a twinge of jealousy?" Halie laughed.

"No – well, yes," Jason said, turning a shade of red.

"That's okay. Kim told me about his place. I've never been there. Maybe we'll get an invitation some day."

"We'd better."

"Hey, I have to get these papers graded," Halie pointed out.

"Can I help you?"

"Sure, it's easy. It's a multiple choice, true-false test. Here's the key," Halie said, as she handed Jason a stack of papers and the test key.

For the next two hours, Jason graded sixth-grade test papers. As he finished his stack, he looked at Halie. She'd been studying him for the last 15 minutes, as he had done her earlier.

"Hey, what's this?" Jason asked.

"I finished a while back. You were concentrating, so I just spent some time looking at you."

"And?"

"You're a very handsome man. You also have great strength in your smile. I can tell by looking at you that you've been through a great deal. I'm just glad you're with me."

Jason reached out for her. She let him guide her to the floor. Pushing papers out of the way, they made love. It was passionate and uninhibited. When they finished, they held on to each other, refusing to pull away.

"Hey, you'd better move those papers before they get ruined."

"Sweetheart, if they're not already ruined, they'll be fine," Halie said, as she kissed him.

The ring of Jason's cell phone broke the silence. It was James. He'd just finished interviewing Al.

"Jason, I need to talk to you. Are you free?"

"Well, actually no, but I can come by in an hour," Jason replied.

"Okay, come to the house. I'll be on the front porch."

Jason was puzzled. It was rare for his father to ask him to come over at night. It was also rare for him to ask that they meet on the front porch. It was clear James didn't want Victoria knowing what they were talking about.

"You're not leaving, are you?" Halie asked.

"Not right now sweetheart. I need to meet my dad in an hour, but

I'll be back. That's, if you want me back."

"I want you to spend the night, Jason. Does that tell you how much I want you to come back?"

"Trust me, I'll be back," he replied. "Besides, we still have another half hour before I have to leave."

"That's plenty of time," Halie said, as she embraced him.

Walking up the front sidewalk, Jason could see his father sitting on the porch. It was past 11:00 p.m. - late for James to be awake.

"Hi, Dad. Sorry I'm so late. I was at Halie's."

"That's okay. How's it going with Halie?"

"Really well. There's something about her that makes me feel good."

"I'm glad for you. I know it's been a tough three years," James commented.

"So, what did you want to talk about?" Jason asked.

"How was your visit with Frederick Menick?"

"Fine. I'm not sure how much he knows. I felt sorry for him."

"Do you think he told you the truth?"

Jason hesitated. He hadn't told James everything about his visit with Frederick.

"I think he did - why?"

"I think he knew the housekeeper. Did he deny meeting any other servants?"

"Yes. He said Oliver never had any servants."

"Hmmm, he lied. I wonder why?" James said aloud.

"Why do you say that?" Jason asked.

"I have my own sources They contradict him," James answered.

"Who?"

"I'm not at liberty to say."

"Wait a minute. You're holding back? I thought we decided to work together on this," Jason commented.

"To a point," James replied.

Jason didn't press. He, too, had withheld information. He hadn't told him about the picture.

"I want to go see Frederick. Will you go with me?" James asked.

"Sure. I can get away around 5:00 p.m. tomorrow. You want me to pick you up?"

"Yes. I'll be waiting," James replied.

Driving back to Halie's apartment, Jason wondered if his father would see the picture that Frederick had in his cabinet. If he did, he'd know he had lied. Neither was willing to open up with the other. Each mistrusted the other's reaction.

Halie had given Jason the key to her apartment. As he climbed into bed next to her, he wondered what his father was thinking. The feel of her body next to him made him forget.

"Hey, handsome. I hope that's you next to me," Halie quipped.

"Yes, it's me. It's good to be here. Don't complain if I snore," Jason laughed.

"I won't. I'm just glad you're here," Halie replied as she turned over to face him.

Jason kissed her. He could feel her body against him. She wrapped her leg around him and squeezed. They fell asleep in each other's arms.

Chapter Thirty-One

Kenny was focused on his computer. Beside him sat a note pad on which he had written down information about Frederick Menick. He closed the computer and hurriedly showered and dressed. Dan and Jane were due to pick him and Melinda up in 10 minutes.

"Kenny, you're always late. Can you, for once, be ready on time?"

"I'm sorry, Melinda. I was just working on what Jason asked me to look into."

"Any luck?"

"Not yet, but I'm not giving up."

Melinda and Kenny lived together. They had for the past six months. They'd set a date for their wedding - immediately following graduation. Melinda's parents had met Kenny and were genuinely happy for her. It didn't take long for Kenny to endear himself. It was his personality. They had been serious when they asked Jason to help them pursue a residency in Chicago. Kenny was still intent on opening a free clinic in the mountains of Western North Carolina. Melinda's parents had pledged financial support. Training in the inner city of Chicago would be beneficial for them both.

Dan and Jane were prompt. At 6:55 p.m., Dan knocked on Melinda's door.

"Hey, Dan, Jane - it's great to see you," Melinda said, as she hugged them.

"Hi, Melinda. You look great," Dan replied.

"Jane, you glad Dan's here?"

"Oh, yeah, at least so far. He hasn't destroyed my house as of yet," she replied.

"Kenny, Dan and Jane are here. You ready?" Melinda called out. "He's worse than a woman, always late."

Melinda showed them in and offered them a glass of wine.

"That would be nice," Jane said as she sat on the couch next to Dan.

"White, if you have it," Dan chimed in.

As Melinda opened the wine, Dan walked over to a grouping of pictures above the desk. Two included Jason and Alyssa getting ready to leave on an outing with other medical students.

"Jane, come here. Look at these pictures."

"Wow - that's Jason and Alyssa. They looked so happy."

"Yeah, I know. Those were better days."

As he turned to go back to the couch, he looked down at the note pad with Kenny's scribbling. The name Frederick Menick was printed on the top of the sheet. *Frederick Menick*, Dan thought to himself. *That's the name of Oliver Conrad's old driver. Why would Kenny be seeking information about him?*

"Thanks, Melinda," Jane said, as Melinda handed Dan and her a glass of wine.

Dan decided not to ask. He had an idea that it had to do with Jason. He knew from his time with him in the cemetery that something was on his mind. Something was going on.

"Kenny, we're glad you could join us," Melinda said sarcastically, as Kenny entered the room.

"Sorry, guys. I've been working on a project. It's my fault. Please accept my apology."

"Not necessary, Kenny. We're enjoying our visit with Melinda," Jane replied.

"Hey, Dan. How's life in Chicago?" Kenny asked.

"It's about the same. Have to always keep my eye on Jason, though. He keeps getting into trouble."

Kenny also wanted to know what Jason was involved in.

"Exactly what kind of stuff is he working on?"

"I don't know," Dan replied, clearly picking up interest in Kenny's voice.

"Bring us up to date on you guys," Jane asked.

"Where do we start?" Kenny replied. "Well, we graduate in May, get married in June, start residency in July. I guess that's about it."

"Kenny, you're something else," Melinda commented. "He leaves the details out - just cuts to the big stuff. First, graduation's on Mother's Day, and we'd love it if you guys could attend. Second, we're getting married on June 5th in Simsbury, Connecticut. We're doing it there because my grandparents live there. I used to spend every summer with them. We're counting on you guys to be at that, too. Finally, we want to do our residencies in Chicago. Kenny's interested in a program at Northwestern, and I'm looking at one at Cook County Hospital, where Jason's dad used to work. Now, that's the detail."

"Thanks, Melinda. I know we'll be at your wedding - count on that. If we can make the graduation, we'll be there too," Jane said, looking at Dan.

"Hey, I wouldn't miss either one for the world," Dan added.

The evening was full of reminiscing. Both couples had come together out of a set of experiences that had ended tragically but had also resulted in loving relationships for each. Halie and Jason were the center of the conversation.

"Tell me more about Halie," Melinda asked.

Dan didn't have much he could add. He hadn't met her. As of yet, Jason hadn't introduced them.

"I wish I could, but all I know is what Jason tells me, what he told Alyssa, and how he acts. What I will say is I think he's really in love. This gal must really be something."

"All we know is she's a teacher, and they met at a party at Jason's house," Kenny responded.

"Actually she teaches at a school just a mile or so from his house. I heard him telling Alyssa on Sunday that she's from Iowa, and her dad's a mail

"So, he still visits Alyssa?" Melinda asked.

"Like clockwork. I brought a six-pack of beer last Sunday. We just sat and talked with Alyssa and each other for a couple hours."

"You took beer into a cemetery?" Jane asked.

"Sure, why not?"

Later, as Dan pulled up in front of Melinda's apartment, he kept wondering what Kenny was working on. Each knew Jason was keeping something secret - something he wasn't willing to divulge even to those closest to him.

"We had a great time, guys. Thanks for dinner," Melinda said.

"We did, too. It was fun," Jane replied.

"So we're going to see you in May and June – right, Dan?" Kenny asked.

"Kenny, I have a feeling you'll see us a lot more before then."

Chapter Thirty-Two

Jackson had completed his autopsy of the remains. There wasn't a great deal to tell. Sitting across from Jason, Claire, and James, he related what he knew.

"First, this baby died at childbirth. Something went wrong while it was in the womb. I can't tell what, but it caused his death," Jackson began.

"His?" James asked.

"Yes, it was a boy."

"Any way to tell how long it's been in the trunk?" Jason asked.

"This is a guess, but, by my count, probably 50 or 60 years. This isn't new. It's been there a long time."

"Any foul play?" Jason pressed.

"No, just a stillborn child," Jackson concluded.

"Well, that's a relief. At least we know someone didn't kill the child. We just need to find out whose child it was and who put him in the trunk," James stated.

Claire and Jackson went back to work. They all agreed to meet at Jason's over the lunch hour. It was the most secure place they knew of. James and Jason stayed behind.

"We still on for this afternoon?" James asked.

"Sure. I'll pick you up."

"Let's just meet here, okay? I don't want Victoria worrying about anything."

"Okay. I'll see you at 5:00 p.m."

Driving back to the precinct, Jason tried to imagine who his father's source could be. It had to be someone from his past. Pulling into a parking place at Precinct 71, he turned off the engine and sat for a moment, thinking about Halie. The night had been perfect. When she kissed him goodbye to go to school, he had felt panic. He thought about the day he said goodbye to

Alyssa for what he thought would only be a few hours. He wished he could protect Halie from anything or anyone who might hurt her. He knew he couldn't. His phone's ring jolted him back to reality. The caller ID told him the call was from Dan.

"Hi, Dan - how's vacation?"

"It's great. We're going out to Carolina Beach today. Thought I'd stop for a minute where Alyssa died. Jane said it would be fine with her. She's quite a woman."

"How was dinner with Melinda and Kenny last night?"

"Fun. They're really happy. They're a funny pair. I think Melinda will rule that household," Dan laughed.

"I know, but sometimes you sacrifice one thing for something else that is of far greater value. Heck, look at you guys - Jane's sacrificing.....," Jason started.

"Okay, I know where you're going with this, so let's drop it," Dan interrupted.

Jason laughed. They knew each other well. They could anticipate what the other one would say.

"Hey, Jason, I need you to be honest about something."

"What?"

"I want to know what's going on. I was at Kenny's last night and saw a piece of paper with Frederick Menick's name on it. I know he was your grandfather's driver. What's Kenny looking into for you?"

Jason hesitated. He had been caught off guard.

"Dan, it's really complicated. I can't talk to you about it over the phone."

"Okay – when, then?"

"When you get back, first thing. Does that work?"

"Yeah, I guess; just be totally honest - alright?" Dan responded.

"I will," Jason replied.

"Tell me at least that you aren't into something that can get you hurt."

"I'm not. That you can believe."

The thought of opening up to Dan was actually a relief for Jason. As he walked into the precinct, he felt better.

The hours at work dragged by. He dreaded taking his father to Frederick Menick's home. His only hope was that Menick had removed the picture. Otherwise, James was sure to notice. Sitting on his porch waiting for his father to arrive, he tried to imagine James's reaction if he saw the picture. He couldn't.

"Hey Dad," Jason said as James walked up the sidewalk.

James had parked along the street. Jason would drive.

"Hi, Jason - you ready?"

"I guess so."

It was a short drive - 15 minutes. Cicero wasn't far from Hinsdale.

"So, this is where Frederick lives?" James said, as they pulled to a stop in front of Menick's home.

"Yep, this is it. Cozy, isn't it?"

"Looks like he held out when the developers put in those apartment buildings."

"He was in your house all through your youth. Seems like you didn't know him very well," Jason remarked.

"I didn't. He was very private, almost a recluse. He never talked about anything. I just thought it was his personality. He and my mom had a good relationship, but, other than that, it was like he didn't live there."

"He lived right above you, yet you didn't know him."

"No, I didn't. I was busy with other things," James responded.

"Did he ever leave the house?"

"Every Sunday afternoon, he'd leave and come back Monday morning. I know, because my mother would always give him a ride to the bus stop."

James and Jason walked up to the front door and knocked.

"Not the best neighborhood," James noted.

"No - pretty shady if you know what I mean," Jason replied.

As they were about to knock again, Frederick answered the door.

"Frederick, it's good to see you," James said to the aging Menick.

"I'll be! James - and Jason; come in."

Walking into the house, Jason scanned the cabinet that had held the picture. It was empty. He felt relieved. The three men took seats in the living room. As before, the small home was neat and tidy.

"James, how are you?" Frederick asked.

"I'm fine. How about you?"

"Good. I got to visit with Jason a couple days ago. That was nice."

"Frederick, I apologize for bringing this up again. I know Jason asked you about it when he visited. Do you remember my father having any servants besides yourself?"

"Well, as I told Jason, no. I was the only one," he replied.

"Do you remember when Al Savuzzo used to come to Oliver's parties?"

"No, your father stopped having parties before I came to work for him," he answered.

Jason was speechless. He'd never heard his father mention the Savuzzo name. He knew Oliver had been part of the Savuzzo family, but his father - it hadn't ever entered his mind. He decided to listen and ask James later.

"When were you hired?" James asked.

"I think it was 1946 or '47 - I'm not sure."

"Did you know Al Savuzzo?"

"Yes, he came over to the house several times."

"What did you do for my father?"

"I did a lot of things. I drove, helped Miriam around the house, did grounds work, ran errands; sometimes, I even babysat with you, James," he responded. "I doubt you remember that."

"Is this where you spent every Sunday night?"

"Yes. My mother and sister lived here."

"What happened to them?"

"My sister moved to New York City 30 years ago. She died of breast cancer in 1988. My mother lived here till she died in 1982," he answered.

"So, who maintained the house? You lived at my father's house until he died, right?"

"Yes, I did. I only wish he hadn't had his stroke on a Monday morning. I might have been able to help."

"And this house," James pressed.

"I came here every Sunday night. I'd work around the house and keep it up."

Jason couldn't understand the track James was on. All he could do was listen. With each question, he learned more and more about his father. He couldn't understand how little his father knew about the man who had lived upstairs from him for more than 20 years.

Chapter Thirty-Three

"Do you know Al Savuzzo?" Jason asked his father on the way back to Jason's house.

James sat silently, looking out the window. He tried to think through how he'd explain knowing Al.

"I met him several times when he used to come to the house. I heard my dad talk about him. He's the only person I knew of who was Oliver's age and still alive."

James quickly changed the subject.

"I just took a wild stab with Frederick. Do you think he was being honest?"

"No. I think he was covering something," Jason answered.

"I agree. He knows something he isn't willing to tell."

"Dad, I should have told you, but, when I was there last time he had a picture of Oliver in front of the '39 Cadillac. It was in the cabinet in the living room. I would swear that, in the background, was an African-American housekeeper."

"Why didn't you tell me this before?"

"I don't know. I just thought I should keep it to myself till we knew more," Jason replied.

"Was it still there?"

"No, he had moved it. I think he may have realized I had gotten a glimpse of it."

James was disappointed in his son. Clearly, he didn't trust him.

"Jason, if we're going to work on this together, you have to be honest with me. We can't hide things from each other."

"You hid the fact that you know Al Savuzzo," Jason replied.

"Yeah, I know, and that wasn't right. Let's call it even and start this over. Deal?"

"Deal," Jason responded. "I need you to know that, when Dan gets back from North Carolina, I'm telling him everything."

"Why?"

"Because he knows I asked Kenny to look into Frederick. There's no way to keep it from him."

"I want to be there when you talk to him. When does he get back?" James asked.

"In three days."

Jason dropped James off at his car and drove around to park his car in the garage. It was 7:00 p.m. He wanted to go by and see Halie, but was reluctant. He didn't want to smother her. He decided instead to call Jeff.

"Jeff - wanna come over and hang out?"

"Sure. Got any beer?" Jeff replied.

"Plenty."

Jason quickly changed and grabbed a bucket, filled it with beer, and poured ice over the top. Sitting in his Adirondack chair, he called Halie.

"Hey, beautiful. How was your day?"

"It was good. The kids were really good for a Thursday. They usually get antsy right before the weekend," she replied. "How was yours?"

"It was interesting. Nothing of substance, but it filled my day," he replied.

"What are you doing tonight?" Halie asked.

"Well, I was going to call to see if I could come see you, but I thought I shouldn't push it, so I called Jeff, and he's coming over."

"Hey, don't ever feel like you're pushing it. I love you being here. You have an open invitation."

"Thanks, sweetheart - I'll remember that," Jason replied. "Unfortunately, I already called Jeff."

"Don't you dare cancel on him. He's your best friend. Enjoy the night. I'll see you tomorrow," Halie responded. "And tomorrow, plan on spending the night, okay?"

"Twist my arm a little more," Jason replied.

"I don't think I have to," Halie laughed.

Jeff arrived just as Jason hung up.

"Have a seat - grab a beer," Jason called out.

"Don't mind if I do," Jeff replied.

"No, Claire's not here. Neither is Meredith," he said, as he noticed Jeff looking around.

"I know that. I was just checking your place out."

Claire and Meredith had always attracted Jeff's attention. Both were beautiful women in very different ways. Claire had a very Italian look, whereas Meredith looked to be Scottish.

"What's up with Meredith? I haven't seen her in a long time," Jeff asked.

"Well, where do I begin? She finishes her residency at Barnes Hospital in St. Louis in three months. She's been hired by a group here in Chicago," Jason started.

"Wow - that means all the Conrads will be together. Bill's still here, right?"

"Oh yeah. He's still with the same cardiology practice. Melanie's pregnant with their third child, which my mom is ecstatic about."

"Yeah, he's the only one producing grandkids," Jeff laughed.

Jason knew all too well that Bill, as usual, had met all the Conrad expectations. Victoria loved being around her grandchildren. They were the focus of her life. Her disappointment that Jason, Claire, and Meredith hadn't produced any was evident. At every family dinner, she would ask when one of them would be giving her another grandchild.

"So, is Meredith seeing anyone?" Jeff asked.

"Funny you should ask. She met a guy during her vacation to Aruba. His name's Michael Grant. I haven't met him, but she seems to be crazy about him."

"He lives in Aruba?"

"No, he was also vacationing there. I think he lives in Orlando, Florida. We don't know much about him. It happened only about a month ago."

"He hasn't visited her?" Jeff asked.

"No, not to my knowledge. They usually meet somewhere. I talked to her last week, and she said she was going to New York City to meet him."

"What's he do for a living?" Jeff pressed.

"No one can really figure that out. I don't even think Meredith knows. All I know is she's hooked," Jason laughed.

Jeff listened intently. For a long time, Jason had thought Jeff had a crush on Claire. He was wrong. Ever since he'd met her at the Conrad home five years before, Jeff had carried a torch for Meredith. Thin, with short, strawberry-blond hair, freckles, and librarian glasses, she never portrayed an image of the kind of woman he ordinarily was attracted to. He never worked up the courage to ask her out, as much because he feared Jason's reaction as because of his own fear of rejection.

"Shouldn't somebody check this guy out to see if he's legit?" Jeff asked.

"I think it's a little early for that. She's been dating him only for a couple months."

"I don't know. He sounds kind of questionable."

For the first time, Jason sensed a real interest in his friend for Meredith.

"Jeff, do I sense jealousy?"

"Okay, I'll admit it. Maybe it's too late, but, yes, I've had a crush on Meredith for a long time. I never told you because I knew you'd make fun," Jeff admitted.

"Wow - I'm sorry. I wouldn't have made fun," Jason replied. "I take that back. Yeah, I would have."

"Well, I just don't want to see her hurt," Jeff remarked.

"Jeff, we have some other stuff going on that's going to have to take priority right now."

"Well with your permission, maybe I'll do it."

"Go ahead," Jason responded. "Let me know if you find anything."

Jason could feel Jeff's concern. He decided that, as soon as something was resolved, he would do a background check on Michael Grant.

Chapter Thirty-Four

Dan enjoyed his week in North Carolina. It lived up to his expectations. Each day, he felt more and more comfortable with Jane. Each day he realized she was his future.

"I enjoyed dinner tonight with Linda," Dan said, as he lay next to Jane in bed.

"Me, too. She's come a long way. She seems genuinely happy."

"Well, meeting Jack Timmons certainly made a big difference."

Linda Phister had fully recovered from her mental breakdown four years before. Now, back at her job, she had met a divorced attorney she'd fallen in love with.

"They make a good couple, don't you think?" Jane asked.

"Yep, I think Linda's going to be just fine."

"Tomorrow's our last day. What do you want to do?"

"I'd like to go the beach again. Let's take some wine, a cooler, and let the sun set behind us as we watch the ocean. What do you say?"

"Sounds great," Jane answered.

Both of them knew they needed to talk about a long-distance relationship. Both had ties to their communities that would be hard to break. It had taken a long time to find each other. They were happy.

As they sat on the beach, drinking wine and watching the sun disappear behind the sand dunes, they were hesitant to bring up the issue. It was a warm, windy day on the beach. The crowds had disappeared, leaving them alone on a wide stretch of sand. Dan poured a glass of wine and held up his glass.

"Here's to a great week with a great woman," he toasted.

Jane smiled and leaned forward to kiss him. As she did, he moved in front of her chair and bent down on one knee.

"Jane Moran, will you marry me and move to Chicago as my wife?"

Dan asked as he pulled an engagement ring from his pocket.

Jane was stunned. She had no idea the proposal was coming. Her mind had been occupied by the thought of who would relocate and whether the relationship would last. At first, she couldn't speak. Tears welled up in her eyes.

"Oh, Dan, you've blown me away. I don't know what to say."

"Say yes. I love you, Jane. You're the most important person in my life. I don't want to waste any more time. Life's too short. Alyssa taught me that."

"I love you, Dan Johnson. Yes, I'll marry you, and yes, I'll move to Chicago. I'm going to freeze my ass off, but you're worth it."

Jane knelt down beside him and kissed him. Dan placed the ring on her finger.

"You've made me so happy," he told her.

"I can't believe this is happening. I had all but given up on the thought of ever finding someone to love again. You changed all that, Dan."

"I wish Alyssa were here today. Right now, this moment - she would've loved it," he said, as he held on to her.

"When did you get the ring?" Jane asked.

"In Chicago, before I left."

"You planned to propose before you left Chicago? How could you be so sure?" Jane asked.

"I know myself. I know when it's right. It felt so good when we were together in Chicago that I decided to ask when I got here."

"Were you the least bit concerned I might say no?"

"That's why I waited till the last night. I figured I'd at least get a great vacation before you turned me down."

Jane smiled.

"You knew I wouldn't turn you down?"

"I knew. I could feel it."

Dan and Jane drank wine and talked until it was dark about wedding plans, the move to Chicago, and when to tell family and friends. Only the full moon reflecting off the ocean gave them light. Holding hands, they walked over the dunes to their car.

"We have so much to do," Jane commented.

"I know. Okay, tomorrow I return to Chicago. Look at your schedule, and see when you can come to Chicago again. We'll plan to get married at that time. Is that okay?"

Jane laughed - she knew there was much more involved.

"Dan, first thing I have to do is put out some feelers for jobs in Chicago."

"Ah, well, I guess I should've told you. I already talked to the Chicago District Attorney. He's an old golfing buddy of mine. I was the best man in his wedding. He has a job for you as an Assistant DA if you want it."

"You must really have been confident," Jane responded. "Lucky I have an Illinois license."

"Are you interested?"

"Sure. Tell him I'll come interview anytime he wants me to."

"Good. Now, tomorrow, let's tell family and friends," Dan replied.

Everything was happening so fast, Jane thought to herself.

The flight back to Chicago went quickly for Dan. It had been a long time since he had thought about the future. Now it was all he could think about. Saying goodbye to Jane at the airport was difficult. Their last kiss was long and passionate. Jane had called her family and friends to tell them about her engagement before he left. Dan would tell them when he got back to Chicago. Jason would be first. It was noon on Sunday when he pulled away from the airport. He knew Jason would be at the cemetery. He planned to tell him there.

Walking up to Alyssa's gravesite, he could see Jason sitting in a lawn chair. Beside him, in another lawn chair, was a pretty, red-haired young woman. Dan knew it was Halie. He was glad Jason had brought her. It was something he needed to do.

"Hey - brought a friend, I see," Dan said, as he placed his chair next to Halie.

"Dan, you're back. That's great. Dan, this is Halie Carson. Halie, this is Alyssa's father, Dan Johnson. Oh, and, by the way, he's my boss."

Halie stood up and offered her hand.

"It's nice to meet you, Mr. Johnson. Jason's told me a great deal about you."

"First, it's Dan, and second, don't believe everything he tells you," Dan laughed.

Halie offered him a beer.

"So, Halie, Jason seems pretty taken with you."

"Well, Dan, I think it's mutual," Halie smiled.

Dan stood up and approached the headstone.

"Alyssa, Jason, Halie, I'm engaged."

Jason looked at Dan and popped open another beer.

"Did I hear you right? Did you say you're engaged? To be married?"

"You heard me right. I asked Jane last night, and I'm sure - much to your surprise - she said yes."

"Whoa - does that mean you're moving to North Carolina?" Jason asked.

"No, it means Jane's going to take a job with the Chicago DA's office."

"She's moving here? Damn, she must really love you," Jason chuckled.

Chapter Thirty-Five

Dan had more to talk about with Jason than just his engagement. He wanted to know what was going on. He knew Jason was working on a case. His gut feeling told him it was related to the Conrad family. He hoped it wasn't centered on James and his visit to Denver.

The visit to the cemetery had gone well. Now, he could put a face to a name for Halie Carson. The conversation beside Alyssa's grave had been honest, forthright, and meaningful. Her supportive, understanding nature made them appreciate who she was.

"Meet me at my house," Jason said to Dan as he helped Halie into his car.

"Okay - 20 minutes?"

"Give me an hour. I need to take Halie home."

"An hour then. See you there," Dan replied.

Halie wondered what was so important that they needed to talk. It was evident they wanted privacy.

"I'm sorry, sweetheart. I just need to talk to Dan about a case. It shouldn't take too long."

"That's okay. Want to come by after you're done?" she asked.

"Yes, if that's okay."

Jason enjoyed spending his free time with Halie. As he opened the car door for her he reached out for her hand. As she got up, she put her arms around him. The kiss was soft and inviting.

"I'll be back as soon as possible," Jason said, as he walked her to the door.

"I hope so. For some reason, I can't get enough of you," she replied.

Dan was waiting on the front porch. He'd taken a seat in one of the Adirondack chairs. Jason laughed as he walked up the porch steps.

"Comfortable, aren't they?"

"Very. Now I know why you come out here to think."

Jason settled into the other chair.

"So, you're getting married?"

"Yep, as soon as possible. Hopefully, Jane can be here in a couple months," Dan replied.

"I'm surprised she agreed to leave the south. She loves it down there."

"Guess she's in love," Dan said, with pride.

"I'm really happy for you, Dan. Couldn't happen to a better person."

"Thanks, Jason."

"I guess we need to talk about why you're here, right?"

Dan smiled. He knew Jason was uncomfortable.

"Jason, just tell me the truth."

Just as Dan finished his sentence, James pulled up in front of the house.

"Dad wanted to be here when I talked to you," Jason said, as he got up from his chair.

"Hi, James," Dan said, as he held out his hand.

"Dan, Jason tells me you're engaged. Congratulations."

"Thanks. Word spreads fast," Dan replied.

"Will you all follow me?" Jason asked.

Jason led them down into the basement. He and James pulled out the trunk.

"What's this about?" Dan asked.

"Sit down Dan."

Dan sat in the pink chair, waiting for Jason to explain.

"Dan, two weeks ago, I came down to the basement and found this trunk. By its marking, it appears to be Oliver's. It had a lock on it that I didn't know how to remove. That's why I used my service revolver two weeks ago. I reported it to the desk sergeant. It took two tries with a hacksaw before I got the lock off."

"Dan, I need to ask you to give us some time to unravel this," James interrupted.

"So, what did you find?"

"We found the skeletal remains of a newborn male child."

Dan sat silently, looking at the trunk. He stood up and moved over to where Jason and James stood.

"Where'd you find the remains?"

"At the bottom, Dan," Jason replied. "It was arranged like a coffin. There were toys, blankets, and clothing. They were all there. On the top was a *Chicago Tribune* from March 18, 1948."

"Do you think the baby was Oliver's?"

"We don't know. We're trying to find out. We asked Jackson to look at the remains to tell us anything he could."

"Jackson - Claire's husband?"

"Yes. He told us the baby died in the womb and was a male. It was stillborn," James responded.

"Why didn't you report this?" Dan asked, looking at Jason.

"Because - it's family. We needed to know more."

"Dan, he wanted to tell you. I pressured everyone to hold back. I take full responsibility," James said.

Dan examined the trunk.

"Do you think there's anything else in the trunk that could help us?" James asked.

"Probably not, but a forensics lab might be able to find something. Tell me what you've done so far."

James and Jason detailed everything that they'd done. They told him about their discussions with Frederick Menick, the search for the housekeeper, and James' visit with Al Savuzzo. They didn't hold back. There was no reason to. If Dan was going to respect their wishes and give them time he needed all the information they had. *Besides*, Jason thought to himself, *he might be able to help.*

"So, now you know everything," Jason said.

"Yeah, guess I do. I'll give you three days. If nothing breaks in three days, we go to the precinct and file a report."

"Thanks, Dan. Can you help us?" James asked.

"I'll do what I can."

The three men climbed the stairs and walked out on to the porch. James said goodbye and drove away. Jason and Dan sat back down in the Adirondack chairs.

"What's your gut tell you?" Dan asked.

"My gut tells me it was the housekeeper's child and that Oliver was the father," Jason answered.

"Who's the key here? Someone's always the key."

"I think it's Frederick Menick."

"Then, let's find out everything we can about him - and I mean *everything.*"

Chapter Thirty-Six

September 1947

Frederick Menick adapted to his new surroundings quickly. Having a home to help care for was important to him. Oliver and Laynie became his extended family. It had been six weeks since he'd been hired by Oliver to serve as a driver and helper for Laynie. Laynie, who objected at first, welcomed the help. It was comforting to have someone in the house when Oliver was gone. Knowing that Frederick was upstairs gave her a safe feeling. For Oliver, it was good to know Laynie wasn't alone.

Six weeks had passed since they'd made love. It had been six weeks of closeness, affection, passion, and caring. It was everything that Oliver had dreamed about in a relationship. For Laynie, it was what she had wanted for years. Watching Oliver consume himself in useless pursuits had taxed her patience. Those memories were gone. Only the happy thoughts of the love they shared existed.

"Oliver, I want you to go to church with me today," Laynie said, as she lay next to him in bed.

"Church - I'm not really comfortable in any church, sweetheart."

"Just this once – please? We have to get out. We can't hide our love forever."

"I know. All right, but I'm not going to say anything. It doesn't matter if it were your church or any other. I'm just not a joiner."

Laynie knew Oliver was skeptical about organized religion. The fact that he had agreed to go to church with her was huge. He hadn't been to church in 15 years.

"Don't be nervous, sweetheart. They won't bite," Laynie said, as they entered Ebenezer Missionary Baptist Church.

Oliver was nervous. He'd never been in a predominantly colored church. His experience with colored people had been limited to Laynie. He had none in his practice or his private life.

"Sorry. I'm just a little out of my element."

"Just listen to the sermon, and pretend to sing. It's just church," Laynie replied.

For the first time in his life, he experienced what it was like to not be White in America. He stood out. He was singular. He was the minority. As much as Laynie tried to comfort him, he felt estranged. Taking their seats in the back of the church, she felt his discomfort.

"If you think this is bad, wait until we go to one of your medical meetings," she whispered.

"I know. I just feel so different," he replied.

The church service was a relief. He didn't have to interface with anyone. Once the service ended, they joined others in line to greet the pastor. Reaching down, he grabbed Laynie's hand.

"Don't leave me. I'm a little scared here," he told her.

"Just relax, Oliver. It'll be okay," she told him, as she squeezed his hand.

Oliver started to sweat. He could feel his collar tighten around his neck. For an instant, he felt dizzy and nauseous. As he neared the pastor, he started to feel relief. He could see the end in sight.

"God bless you," Reverend Silas Thompson said as he shook Oliver's hand.

"Thank you," Oliver replied.

"It's a pleasure having you with us today," Silas continued.

"I loved your sermon, Reverend Thompson," Laynie said.

"Thank you, Laynie. It's great seeing you."

As they walked down the steps of the church, Oliver felt hundreds of eyes on him. Laynie held on to him. She knew he was uncomfortable. With each step, she gained an appreciation for who he was. He'd ventured outside his comfort zone. He knew what was waiting. As they walked back to the bus stop, she pulled him close.

"Thank you, sweetheart."

"Why?" he asked.

"Because I know that had to be difficult. I know how uncomfortable it was for you. You knew it would be and still came. I admire you," Laynie replied.

"Hey, I love you. I know we have a rough road ahead. I'm willing to work through it."

Laynie appreciated Oliver's sentiment, but she also knew the real test for him would come from his own community. Frederick was waiting for them when they got home.

"Dr. Conrad, Laynie, did everything go okay?"

"Frederick, will you call me Oliver? If you don't, I'm going to have to fire you."

"Oliver, you will do no such thing," Laynie scolded.

"No, but please call me Oliver."

"Yes, sir. Oliver, did everything go okay?" Frederick asked again.

Frederick had begun to think of Oliver and Laynie as his family. He would protect them, no matter what.

"It was a bit uncomfortable, but he did great Frederick," Laynie answered.

"I'm glad."

Sunday afternoons for Oliver and Laynie were relaxed and informal. Most of the day was spent on the front porch. If Oliver wasn't sitting next to her, discussing world events, he was working on his Cadillac. During the week, his life was full of work. At nights and on weekends, he focused on Laynie. They settled into a pattern. It was the most fulfilling relationship he'd ever been involved in. As long as they stayed private, no one judged. Attending Laynie's church was easy in Oliver's mind. Taking her to a hospital medical meeting was something else entirely.

Chapter Thirty-Seven

It was the cramping and nausea that gave Laynie the first hint. Sitting at the kitchen table, she couldn't deny the signs. At first, the missed period was explainable. She had had times in her life when her periods were irregular. But, when she started to feel tired, began to experience nausea, and felt a change in her breasts, she feared what she knew. She was pregnant.

"Are you okay?" Frederick asked.

"I'm fine, Frederick, just a little tired."

Frederick knew Laynie was pregnant. It wasn't difficult to see the changes and surmise her condition.

"Please excuse my forwardness - but are you with child?" he asked.

Laynie hesitated. Even Oliver hadn't picked up on the signs.

"Frederick, can I trust you?"

"Yes, with your life."

Laynie trusted him. She didn't hesitate to tell him that she thought she was going to have a baby.

"Dr. Conrad will be happy."

"I don't know, Frederick. I just don't know."

"I'm sure he will be. I would be."

Without hesitancy, Laynie opened up. She felt safe with Frederick. She had no fear that he'd hurt her. It didn't matter if he judged her. She needed the release. Luckily, he cared, genuinely cared, about her.

"You haven't told Dr. Conrad yet?" Frederick asked.

"No, I don't know how."

"Just be honest. He's in love with you. He'll understand."

"I just don't want to hurt him," she replied.

Except for the attendance at her church, no one except Frederick knew they were together. She would start to show soon. People would know.

"Laynie, it's going to be a while before you start to show. Maybe, during that time, you can open up with Dr. Conrad."

"I think I have to tell him now," she replied.

"It would be best. You have some time if you want to wait."

Oliver's last patient was scheduled at 4:30 p.m. It was 5:30 p.m. by the time he got into his car to drive home. He knew Laynie would be waiting. He smiled as he anticipated the hug and glass of lemonade she would give him as he walked in the back door. He would sit down on a chair at the kitchen table and tell her about his day, as she rubbed his shoulders. The smells that came from what she was cooking for dinner would awaken his taste buds.

"Wow - that smells good. What are you cooking?" he asked, as he turned and kissed Laynie's hand.

"That's Beef Stroganoff. I know you like it."

"I think I like everything you make."

"That's just because you love me," Laynie laughed.

"What did you do today, babe?" Oliver asked.

"The usual - clean, arrange, pick up, launder, etc. etc.," she responded.

"Is Frederick around?"

"He's upstairs."

"Is he working out?" Oliver asked.

"Oliver, hiring Frederick was brilliant. He's a very nice, respectful man who isn't afraid of work. It's nice knowing someone is here when you're gone," she replied. "Go ahead - say you told me so."

Chuckling Oliver pulled her on to his lap.

"I told you so, sweetheart."

Laynie held on tightly. She knew she had to tell him.

"Oliver, I have something I need to tell you," Laynie started.

"You're going to have a baby, aren't you?"

"How did you now?"

"Laynie, I'm a doctor. I notice things. I heard you in the morning in the bathroom. I noticed the sensitivity of your breasts. I just had a gut feeling."

"Why didn't you say something?"

"Because, I felt like you'd come to me when you were ready."

Laynie kissed his forehead and put her head against his chest.

"Oliver.....," she began.

"You don't need to say anything. We're going to have a baby. I'm going to be a father," he responded.

Laynie began to cry - not out of loss or despair but out of love. She hadn't expected the kind of understanding that he was showing. She scolded herself quietly that she hadn't had faith in him and in their love.

Chapter Thirty-Eight

Five months had passed. Laynie and Oliver had yet to venture out into Oliver's world. They'd kept their relationship secret. Only Frederick knew the truth. Laynie was now showing. She limited her trips to those that were absolutely necessary. Frederick did the shopping, ran the errands, and made sure she was protected. Oliver went to work each day and retreated to their home at night. His only absence was due to nights he was on call or when Al Savuzzo needed his services.

Since she'd told him about the pregnancy, he'd been supportive. He'd done everything to make her feel loved and secure - everything but propose. With each day, she wondered if he had the courage. The longer it went, the more she wondered.

"Frederick, do you think Oliver will marry me?" Laynie asked.

"Laynie, I don't know what Dr. Conrad will do. I know he loves you. Whether he can take the step, I don't know."

"Neither do I," she replied. "I love him, and I don't want to hurt him. I fear being with me will do that."

"Oh, Laynie, don't anticipate the worst. Give him a chance."

"Look at me, Frederick - I'm showing. It's pretty clear I'm pregnant. You and Oliver make sure I stay in the house. You've even bought baby clothes and toys for me. I don't like being holed up."

Frederick knew Laynie was starting to doubt whether Oliver could go through with the relationship. It was apparent that he didn't want to make it public. Although he'd espoused his commitment to her, he'd begun to waiver. He loved her. That wasn't the question. Living each day as a couple with a child was. He didn't say anything, but Frederick knew what was in his mind. He knew the birth of the child would put extraordinary pressure on them.

"Hi, Oliver," Laynie said, as he walked in the back door.

Oliver set his medical bag down and walked over to her.

"How's the little one today?" he asked.

"Good. She kicked today. Pretty strong right leg."

Placing his hand on her stomach, he waited for the baby to kick.

"Must be taking a late nap."

"She'll wake up soon. I've made meatloaf for dinner. Is that okay?"

"Sure. You know I love meatloaf. Did you make mashed potatoes?"

"Yes, and a chocolate cake for dessert."

The evening went as so many had for the past five months. There was warm conversation, genuine caring, and mutual desire. The subject of future commitment never came up. Oliver made sure of that.

Laynie went to bed early. She was tired. Oliver poured himself a glass of brandy and sat down in his favorite chair in the den. It was cold in Chicago. Highs during the day barely reached 10 degrees. Frederick had started a fire, knowing Oliver would eventually be in the den. Looking into the fire, Oliver thought about his life. He was torn. The fear of community response made him hesitant to commit.

"Why are you so afraid?" he said aloud to himself.

"What's more important, being with the woman you love or what other people think?" he continued.

The choice wasn't simple. Although he loved Laynie, he knew his career could be in jeopardy if their love became public. Years growing up as a Conrad made him hold back. He knew she was waiting for an outward display to the public of his love for her. He couldn't take the step. He hated himself for his weakness. As much as he loved her, he couldn't act.

"Frederick, you have a minute?" Oliver asked, as Frederick walked by the den.

"Yes, sir, of course."

"Frederick, you've been part of this household for nearly six months. I need your advice."

Frederick sat down opposite Oliver in front of the fireplace.

"I don't know what to do. I love Laynie. You know that. I just can't get myself to act."

"Why?" Frederick asked.

"I don't know. Yes, I do. I'm just afraid of what people will say. I don't want to lose my practice. I fear the backlash if we went public, especially with a baby."

"Dr. Conrad, Laynie's a wonderful woman. She's going to give you the greatest gift possible, a child. All she asks in return is your love. Don't lose the best thing that could ever happen to you."

"I know. It's just so complicated."

Sitting on the stairs, unknown to Oliver and Frederick, was Laynie. She heard it all. Hearing Oliver's hesitancy only confirmed what she knew in her heart. He wasn't strong enough to declare his love for her and her baby.

"Dr. Conrad, er Oliver, don't let this end. She loves you. I know you love her. Excuse me for saying this, but she's the most beautiful woman I've ever seen. What's so amazing about her is she doesn't know how beautiful she is. She's more beautiful inside than she is outside."

"I know, Frederick. I'm lucky she loves me."

"Yes, you are - very lucky. I'd do anything for someone like Laynie," Frederick replied.

As Frederick spoke a tear trickled down Laynie's cheek.

Chapter Thirty-Nine

Al Savuzzo walked up the sidewalk to Oliver's home. Bruno Caseo had driven by a week before and had seen a pregnant Laynie walking down the sidewalk to get the mail. Frederick saw him coming. He guessed who he was. Beside Al walked Caseo. Before they got to the door, Frederick met them.

"May I help you?"

"Yeah, tell Oliver Al's here. We'll wait out here."

Oliver was in the den, Laynie in the kitchen.

"Oliver, Al Savuzzo's outside. He's asking for you."

Oliver felt dread. The only reason Al would visit would be if he knew about Laynie. Someone had seen her. It had been seven months. The fact that it stayed hidden for that long was beyond what he expected.

"Hey, Al, to what do we owe this pleasure?"

"Don't bullshit me, Oliver. Bruno tells me your housekeeper's gonna have a kid."

"What are you talking about?"

Frederick walked into the kitchen. He didn't want Laynie hearing the conversation or walking out on to the porch while Al was there.

"Laynie, stay in here. Al Savuzzo's on the porch."

"He is? Is Oliver talking to him?"

"Yes. Savuzzo and his bodyguard are out there."

Laynie wanted to know what was being said.

"Bring her out here. We'll see for ourselves," Al insisted.

"No, I won't do that. Yes, she's pregnant with my child."

Al and Bruno were stunned.

"Your kid - she's gonna have your kid?" Al asked.

"Yes. Is that so surprising?"

Al looked at Bruno.

"He's expecting a kid - and a colored kid at that," Al said, laughing.

Bruno smiled. He rarely spoke for fear of saying the wrong thing. He was Al's muscle. Although he felt he owed Oliver for mending his gunshot wound, he knew who his boss was. Frederick was listening just inside the door. He wanted to be close at hand in case something happened. Laynie waited in the kitchen. She feared a confrontation would take place.

As Al and Bruno drove away, Oliver walked back inside.

"Everything okay, Oliver?" Frederick asked.

"It's fine. They're gone. I don't think they'll be back."

"Oliver, everything okay?" Laynie asked, as she walked in from the kitchen.

"Yes. It was Al and Bruno. Bruno saw you last week. I told them about us and that we're thrilled to be looking forward to being parents."

"Will this be trouble for you?"

"No. It's none of their damned business, anyway."

Laynie sighed and reached out for his hand.

"You know, maybe we need to start using the back porch more. I'm not sure it's too smart to be going public yet," Oliver said, as he held her hand.

"You really feel that way?" Laynie asked.

"Yes. I think so."

Oliver couldn't read the disappointment that Laynie felt.

"I can't stay holed up here like I'm in jail, Oliver."

"It's just till the baby's born."

On Monday morning, Oliver left early to prepare for morning surgeries. The exchange with Al and Bruno was still on his mind. He didn't care that Al knew he had fathered a child with Laynie, but he feared it might get out to others. Frederick left around 9:00 a.m. to go to the grocery store. Laynie sat alone in the kitchen, nursing a cup of coffee. Surprisingly, it was a mild day in Chicago. The sun brought the temperatures up to the mid-'50s, and, without any appreciable wind, it was tolerable. Setting down her coffee cup, she walked up the stairs and changed into a dress. She felt like getting out. It had been too long.

"I think it's time I got out more often," she said aloud to herself.

Picking out a blue plaid maternity dress, she put on flats and picked a coat out of the coat closet. Her feet were swelling each day, and only flats were comfortable enough to wear.

"Okay – now, where do I want to go?"

She decided to take the bus to her church. She felt comfortable there. People knew her. Hinsdale was a white community. Blacks walking down the sidewalk were assumed to be servants. Two blocks from the Conrad home, she passed a home occupied by one of Oliver's partners in his medical practice, Dr. Stillwell Jordan. She remembered Oliver pointing it out six months before, when they were on their way to church. Since then, she hadn't ventured outside the house or the yard. As she walked by, she could see Mrs. Jordan standing in the window, watching passersby. Laynie waved; Mary Jordan waved back.

"She must wonder what a pregnant colored woman is doing walking in front of her house," she chuckled to herself.

Mary Jordan watched her as Laynie stopped to cross the street.

"Laynie, what are you doing out?" Frederick called out as he stopped in front of the Jordan house.

"I'm going to church."

Laynie walked over to the car. Frederick leaned out and asked her to get in.

"No, I need the walk."

As they talked, Mary Jordan watched. She recognized Frederick as Oliver's driver. He'd driven Oliver to several medical events that she'd attended.

"Please get in, Laynie. I'll take you wherever you want to go," Frederick pleaded.

"I want to go to my church in Cicero."

"Okay, I'll take you there. I'll even show you where my mother and sister live."

Frederick got out of the car and walked around to where she was standing. He opened the back door.

"Let me be your driver today - okay?"

"If you insist," Laynie replied, as she took his hand.

The exchange didn't go unnoticed.

"Why did Oliver's driver pick up a pregnant colored woman?" Mary said to herself. "Why would she sit in the back seat as if he were her driver?"

Chapter Forty

The drive to Ebenezer Baptist took 15 minutes. When they pulled up in front, Laynie asked Frederick to wait in the car.

"It won't take long. I just want to see if Reverend Silas is in."

"I'll be here if you need me," Frederick replied, as he opened the back door.

On the steps to the church were two older women. Frederick and Laynie weren't over-looked. A pregnant colored woman being driven around by a white driver wasn't the norm in Cicero, Illinois. It took only a few minutes to get to the church offices. Silas Thompson was studying the Bible as Laynie knocked gently on the door.

"Laynie, come in. I was just starting to prepare next Sunday's sermon."

"Reverend Silas, I don't want to disturb you," Laynie replied.

"Nonsense - you aren't. Now sit down and tell me what's going on in your life. From the looks of it, you'll be bringing into the world another one of God's children in the near future."

"Yes, I'm due in March."

"I haven't seen you in church lately. Is that why?"

"Partly," Laynie responded. "Reverend Silas, I need your advice."

"That's what I'm here for," he smiled.

"Remember Oliver Conrad? He came to church with me six months ago."

"Yes. He seems to be a fine gentleman," Silas replied. "Is he the father?"

"Yes."

"Are you in love with him?"

"Yes, very much so," she answered. "My fear is that he wants to keep our relationship secret."

"Interracial marriages offer up their own unique challenges, Laynie. Are you ready to meet those challenges?"

"Yes. I think I am, but we haven't even talked about marriage. I think Oliver's afraid."

Silas scratched his head.

"Do you blame him?"

"I know he's thinking about what going public would do to his practice, let alone marriage," Laynie replied.

"Laynie, if you love him and want this relationship, talk to him. Tell him how you feel. As a couple, you can't hide forever. What's he said about the baby?"

"He says he wants to be a father - no matter what."

"Don't force him to take a step. That never works. He has to want to because he loves you. Talk to him. Tell him what's in your heart. You're the only one who can decide what kind of life you want," Thompson advised.

"Thank you, Reverend Silas. This has helped."

"See you in church soon?"

"Yes, you will," Laynie replied.

"God bless you, Laynie. Remember, God loves you."

Laynie knew she had to confront Oliver. She had to let him know what she was feeling. She hoped he would understand and that they could move forward together.

"You okay?" Frederick asked, as Laynie got in the car.

"Yes, it was good to come today. I needed to talk to Reverend Silas. He always seems to show me what I need to do."

"I'm glad. Would you like to see where I live?" Frederick asked.

"Yes, but you live with us, don't you?"

"I do, but I mean where I lived before I moved in with you and Oliver."

The drive to Grand Boulevard took 5 minutes. They parked in front of Frederick's house. For the next 10 minutes, they talked about his mother.

"Your mother and sister still live here?" Laynie asked.

"Yes. I come every Sunday night and help them around the house. It's really small. It's nice to have some room now."

"Oliver told me about what you all went through in Germany. It had to be very difficult."

"Laynie, they were bad days - days I'd like to forget. My mother's a strong woman. She's been there for my sister and me through everything."

"Can I meet them?" Laynie asked.

"You really want to?"

"Yes, I do."

Frederick helped her out of the car and held her arm as they walked up the sidewalk. As he opened the door he called out.

"Mama, it's Frederick - are you home? I have someone I'd like you to meet."

Gertrude Menick dried her hands and came out of the kitchen. She was a short, overweight woman in her mid-'50s. Her eyes showed the pain she'd experienced and the suffering she'd seen. At the same time, they showed strength.

"Frederick, I'm not dressed. I'm so sorry. He should know better," Gertrude said as she shook Laynie's hand.

"Mama, this is Laynie Jessup. She and Dr. Conrad are my employers."

"It's very nice to meet you. Frederick speaks very well of you and Dr. Conrad."

"Thank you, Mrs. Menick. We think a lot of your son. You should be very proud of how you raised him."

Gertrude believed in formality. Appropriateness was extremely important. She was also a warm, genuine person. Frederick and his sister Rita were her life.

"Please sit down, Miss Jessup. Can I get you a cup of tea?"

"That would be nice," Laynie replied.

"Frederick, go get your sister. She's in the back yard."

Rita Menick's auburn hair and olive complexion were in stark contrast to Frederick. She was a beautiful woman. Laynie was taken aback by her looks.

"Hi, my name's Rita. You must be Laynie."

"Yes, I am. It's nice to meet you."

Both Rita and Gertrude spoke English fluently, with a slight German accent. Rita had found employment with a law firm as a legal aid. Gertrude maintained the home. As Gertrude served tea, the four sat in the living room and got to know each other. The Menicks were a close-knit family. They were protective of each other.

"Laynie, when are you due?" Rita asked.

"In March. I'm tired of being pregnant," she replied.

"Dear, it'll be over before you know it, and then you'll miss it," Gertrude responded.

Frederick had little to say. He sat quietly as his mother, sister, and Laynie talked about the impending birth. It was clear they got along well. Laynie felt a refreshing acceptance and hospitality. Before long, three hours had passed. Looking over at Frederick, Laynie noticed he was asleep.

"I guess our talk bored him," she noted.

"Laynie, Frederick can fall asleep anywhere, anytime," Rita commented.

"He's a wonderful man, Mrs. Menick. You both should be proud. There's such a caring spirit in him."

"Thank you. He's had a lot to shoulder since his father and brothers died. I don't know what we'd do without him."

Laynie walked over to the couch and tapped Frederick on the shoulder.

"Oh, I'm sorry. You ready to go?" he asked.

"I think we'd better," Laynie replied. "It's getting late."

Rita and Gertrude were already standing by the door.

"Mama, Rita, I'm sorry I fell asleep. Please forgive me."

Rita laughed.

"Frederick, it's nothing new. You always fall asleep."

Laynie hugged each of them.

"Thank you," she whispered in Gertrude's ear.

"You're welcome here anytime," Gertrude replied.

Rita waved as they drove away. She sensed that her brother felt more for Laynie than just friendship. She knew he was slow to express emotion. The look on his face as he had introduced Laynie told her how much he cared for her.

"Mama, I think our boy is smitten," Rita told her mother.

"What are you talking about?"

"Did you see how he looked at her?"

"I guess not. What do you mean?" Gertrude asked.

"I think he loves her."

Laynie had been silent for the first five minutes of the drive back to Hinsdale. She still felt the warmth of the Menick family.

"Frederick, you have a wonderful family. You're so lucky," Laynie said, as she watched the houses of Cicero go by.

"Thank you, Laynie. They're really good people. I'm glad you got to meet them."

"Your sister is beautiful. She looks so different from you."

"She looks like my father. I look like my mother. In Germany, you either have fair complexion like me, or you have olive skin like Rita. Sometimes people think she's Italian."

It was 3:30 p.m. As they turned the corner to their street, they saw Oliver's car parked out front.

"Oh, no. Oliver's home. He wasn't supposed to be home for another hour."

"Don't worry - he'll understand. I'll explain," Frederick said, as he pulled into the driveway.

Chapter Forty-One

Present Day

Jason brought beer and potato chips out to the porch. He offered them to Dan.

"So you're sure the woman you saw in the picture at Frederick's house was the housekeeper?" Dan asked.

"I'm sure it was. There isn't any other explanation."

"Nothing yet from Kenny?"

"No - he said it would be tough," Jason replied. "He suggested we look for the church she attended. He thinks she would've walked to the bus station and that she would've found a Black church close to where she got off."

"Have you pulled the 1947 CTA schedule?" Dan asked.

"No, I'm going to do that tomorrow."

"Good. I'll do a background check on Frederick. We need to know all we can about him."

Jason had been reluctant to talk to Dan about the pictures that were missing. He feared that his father was involved with the Savuzzo family.

"Hey, can you show me that picture of your dad you told me about?" Dan asked, as he rose from the Adirondack chair.

"That's the thing Dan, it's missing. I think my dad took it when he looked at the pictures a few nights ago."

Dan was relieved. He knew it most likely was Anthony Savuzzo. James was protecting Jason. He didn't want him to know he'd been involved with his best friend's business.

"Let's focus on the baby first, okay?" Dan suggested. "We can always come back to those pictures later."

"Okay, if you think that's wise."

"Sure. Now you need to go see a young lady," Dan replied.

Jason had been gone for almost two hours. He had lost track of time. As he knocked on the door he expected Halie to be gone.

"Hey, Jason - long conversation, wasn't it?" she asked opening the door.

"Yes, I'm sorry. You're going to dump me before long as many times as I'm late."

"No," Halie laughed. "I figure if you're late, there has to be a good reason."

"Thanks, sweetheart. I got involved in bringing Dan up to date on this case. It just took longer than I thought it would."

Halie wrapped her arms around his neck and kissed him. Each time she hugged him, she always added a squeeze at the end. To Jason, it was like saying, "I love you."

It was 3:15 p.m. Jason's mind kept going over what he and Dan had discussed.

"Halie, would you mind if we went on a ride?" Jason asked.

"No - where're we going?"

"Cicero."

Plenty of daylight remained. Jason had no plan, only to drive around. He didn't know what he'd find, but he felt compelled to try. He decided to start at Frederick Menick's home and move out, block by block.

"I really appreciate this, sweetheart," Jason said as he drove past Menick's home.

"Kind of a depressing neighborhood," Halie commented.

"I know. I think at one time it wasn't too bad. It went downhill in the '70s."

For the next hour, they drove around Cicero. Jason was searching - searching for an African-American church near a bus stop. At 5:15 p.m., just as the heat of the day was at a peak in Chicago, he saw it - a deserted church a block from a CTA bus stop. An old sign identified it as Ebenezer Missionary

Baptist Church. He pulled over to the side of the road, pulled out a flashlight, and got out of the car. Halie joined him.

"Is this what you're looking for?" Halie asked.

"Yes, it is," Jason replied as he walked over to the sign.

Written in block letters was the name "Reverend Silas Thompson, Jr."

"I wonder how long this church has been empty?" Halie asked.

"I don't know, but it looks like a good while."

Together, they walked up to the front door. Weeds covered the area in front and grew between the concrete steps. All the windows had been boarded up. Scrap metal and lumber pieces sat spread out over the side yard. Jason pushed on the front door.

"Jason, should you be doing that?"

"Hey, I'm a cop. Arrest me," he laughed.

Two hard shoves forced the door open. Turning on the flashlight, he walked inside.

"Why don't you stay here? I'll be right back," he told her.

"Ah, no. I'm right behind you."

Slowly, they walked through the main sanctuary of the church. Pews had been stripped and removed. The altar was gone. The church had been gutted.

"I have a feeling this is the place," Jason said aloud.

"What did you say?" Halie asked.

"Nothing - just trying to imagine someone being here 60 years ago."

The church, located only five minutes from Frederick's house, had to be the housekeeper's church, Jason thought to himself. Getting back in the car, he sat for a moment and tried to visualize a time when it was active and alive.

"Would you mind if I make a call, sweetheart?" Jason asked.

"No, go ahead. I'm getting intrigued by all this."

As they pulled away from the church, he dialed Dan's number.

"Dan, I think I found the church. I can't explain it, but I think it's the one."

"Is it still operating?"

"No, looks like it closed years ago. I have a name that might tell us where they went," Jason replied.

"What name?" Dan asked.

"Silas Thompson, Jr. I think he was the pastor."

"Okay, we have our work cut out. Good job. What happened with Halie?" Jason hesitated.

"Well, actually, she came with me."

"Jason, you know better than to do that. Don't ever involve a civilian in an investigation. It's too dangerous."

"I know. It was a mistake. It won't happen again."

Halie could tell he was getting reprimanded. She knew most likely it was because she was with him.

"I get you in trouble?" she asked.

"No, not at all. I brought you. It wasn't your fault."

On their way home they drove past Frederick's home again. He was outside, sitting on one of the lawn chairs. He looked sad. He looked up just as they drove by. He recognized Jason and waved. Jason waved back.

Chapter Forty-Two

James was frustrated. He wanted answers, yet all he had were questions. Sitting at his dining room table, eating dinner, he wondered what Jason and Dan would find. He feared the worst. Amidst the investigation, he also worried about his family finding out about his relationship with Anthony Savuzzo.

"You seem lost in thought, James," Victoria observed.

"I'm sorry. I was thinking about Jason. I'm glad he's found someone," James replied.

"I hope he brings her over for dinner soon."

"Why don't you call him and ask?"

"I will - that's a good idea," Victoria responded.

After dinner James sat at his desk and pulled out the pictures of him with Anthony. He slowly, deliberately, tore them into little pieces and discarded them in the trashcan.

"No one can ever know," he said aloud to himself.

The doorbell brought him back from deep thought. It was Claire and Jackson.

"Hi Claire, Jackson - what brings you by tonight?"

"We just wanted to talk a little. Can you come outside? Mom doesn't need to hear this." Claire replied.

"Sure," James said, as they took seats on the porch.

"Dad, Jason called me today and said you talked to Dan. Is that right?"

"Yes, Jason couldn't hold back anymore. Dan said he'd help us, but, in three days, he would have to treat it officially," James replied.

"Dan's going to help?"

"Yes."

"Dad, Jackson and I think we should check the DNA of the remains against Grandfather's," Claire suggested.

"I figured that was why you were here. You want to use mine to see if we're related, right?"

"Yes. I'm sorry, but we'll know for sure then."

James looked at Jackson.

"So what do you need - a swab, skin scraping, hair sample?"

"Well, actually, I'd like all three," Jackson responded.

"Then let's get it done."

It only took a few minutes, and Jackson had what he needed.

"How long will it take to get the results?"

Jackson looked at the samples.

"A day or two. I'll call you when we have the results."

"Better yet, let's all meet at Jason's house. Text me when it's ready, and I'll set up the meeting," Jason replied.

"Hi, Mom," Claire said, as she saw Victoria coming out the door.

"I didn't know you were here."

"We just came by to say hi," Claire replied.

"So, how're you all doing?" Victoria asked.

Claire and Jackson had come by to see James and Victoria for another reason.

"Actually, Mom and Dad, I'm pregnant," Claire announced.

"I knew it," Victoria said, as she reached out and hugged her daughter.

"Congratulations," James said, shaking Jackson's hand.

"Well, now at least Bill can't claim to be the only Conrad to give you a grandchild," Claire laughed.

"Have you told anyone else?"

"No, you're the first. We'll call everybody else today," Jackson answered.

"Claire, when's the baby due?"

"In April - maybe I can hit your birthday, Mom."

"That would be nice," Victoria replied.

James and Victoria spent the rest of the evening sitting on the front porch, talking. It was mid-August, and the air was thick and warm. Even so, it was pleasant on the porch. A slight breeze gave them air.

"James, looks like we're going to add number four to our list of grandchildren," Victoria said smiling.

"Yes, that was good news. I'm glad Claire and Jackson got back together. I always thought they made a good couple."

"We've been fortunate with our children. They've all done well. I hope Jason and Halie are permanent."

"He seems to be in love," James responded.

"I'm worried about Meredith," Victoria replied.

"Meredith - why?"

"I don't know about this Michael Grant she's seeing. No one seems to know anything about him, not even Meredith."

Neither James nor Victoria had met Grant. Meredith spoke in glowing terms about how he'd built her confidence, made her feel respected, and helped her see the people around her in a different light. Every time she spoke about Grant, it was easy to see she was in love. At the same time, any questions about who he was fell on deaf ears. Meredith preferred to talk only about his positive effect on her life.

"I'm sure he's fine. Meredith wouldn't be with someone who was questionable," James replied.

"James, do you know how good some of these guys can appear? I'm sure once he found out Meredith was a doctor, his ears perked up. I'm just a little suspicious."

Chapter Forty-Three

It only took 24 hours for Jane to connect with Josiah Harris. As the District Attorney for the Cook County District Attorney's office, he had the power to hire and fire Assistant DAs. Dan Johnson had highly recommended Jane for a job. After a phone interview, Harris asked that she come to Chicago for a personal interview. The flight from Wilmington arrived on time.

"Jane, over here," Dan called out as she walked off the escalator.

"Hi, Dan. I don't have any luggage," Jane told him. "I carried on."

"Great, let's go, then. My car is at the curb. I can usually get away with about 15 minutes, but that's about all," he laughed. "First, can a guy kiss his fiancée?"

He kissed her before she could answer. Within minutes, they were driving away from the O'Hare International Airport.

"You said on the phone your interview's at 3:00 p.m., right?" Dan asked.

"Yes, with the senior ADA," Jane replied.

"Who is the senior ADA, anyway?"

"Her name's Lisbeth Williams. Josiah Harris is really impressed with her work. Apparently, she's really smart and very successful. I think her conviction ratio is 97%. That's amazing."

"Hey, they'll be lucky to get you. I'd put you up against anyone."

"Thanks, sweetheart, but I think you're partial. So, have we set a date yet?" Jane asked.

"Soon, very soon," Dan replied, as he pulled up in front of the County Clerk's office.

"What're we doing here?"

"Marriage license, babe," he answered.

"Ah - good plan," Jane said smiling.

It was 11:00 a.m. Jane still had four hours before her interview. She'd spend the night and return to Wilmington in the morning.

"Lunch?" Dan asked after they had finished filling out the appropriate forms for the license.

"Sure, where?"

"Downtown Dawg. Best in the world."

Jane laughed. She enjoyed Dan's sense of humor and sense of surprise. As they drove downtown, Dan's cell phone rang. It was Victoria Conrad.

"Hi, Victoria - to what do I owe this pleasure?"

"Dan, first: congratulations. Jason tells me you're engaged."

"Thank you, and, yes, I am, to the most beautiful woman in the world," Dan replied, as he winked at Jane.

"Where are you having the ceremony?"

"Well, we haven't decided yet. Jane's sitting next to me. She has an interview with the Chicago DA this afternoon. If we're lucky, she might have a job before sunset."

"Can I talk to her?"

"Sure," Dan replied, as he handed the phone to Jane. "She wants to talk to you."

Jane took the cell phone from Dan's hand.

"Hello, Mrs. Conrad; this is Jane Moran."

"Call me Victoria - and congratulations. Jason told me the news."

"Thank you, Victoria."

"I know you don't know me all that well, but I'd like to offer our home for your wedding. I think it would be a wonderful place to get married."

"Wow - that's really nice. Let me talk to Dan. I'll call you back tonight. Would that be alright?" Jane asked.

"That would be great, Jane. Again, congratulations."

Jane handed the phone back to Dan.

"What was that about?" he asked.

"The Conrads want us to have the wedding in their home."

"Really. What do you think of that?"

"I've never been to their home. What's it like?"

"It's huge. I liken it to a castle. It would be a good place. They really took Alyssa and me into their family."

"This is going to be just family and a few close friends – right, Dan?"

"Right. That's all I want."

"Let's talk after the interview, okay?"

"Sure," Dan replied, as he pulled up in front of the Cook County Courthouse.

"Wish me luck," Jane said, as she opened the door.

Dan leaned over and kissed her.

"Good luck, babe. Knock 'em dead. See you in an hour."

Prior to picking Jane up at the airport, Dan had ordered a full background check on Frederick Menick. The news from Jason about the church and Silas Thompson was encouraging. Jason would follow the Thompson lead. He would work on Menick. When he got back to the precinct, the report on Menick was in. As he scanned the report, he tried to pick out any irregularity or issue. There was none. Menick had led a quiet, law-abiding life. Other than the home in Cicero, he had had no other addresses. Oliver Conrad had been the only person he'd ever worked for. A check of bank records indicated very little. The only item of interest was a regular $1,000-a-month cash deposit made to Frederick's account. It wasn't salary, as salary was identifiable on the bank statement. The deposit would always be on the first Monday of the month and had started in 1952. The deposits ended in 1999.

Before he finished reading the entire report, Dan realized the hour had ended, he needed to pick up Jane.

"Hey - sorry I'm a little late," Dan apologized.

"No problem. I just finished anyway."

"How'd it go?"

"It went great. I think Lisbeth Williams really liked me."

"What's she like?" Dan asked.

"She's very intelligent, really attractive, and extremely focused on her job."

"When will you hear something?"

"Dan, they offered me the job today. Josiah Harris talked with Lisbeth for a few minutes after the interview and then came out and made me an offer."

"Wow! Did you take it?"

"Yes, I did. I start in four weeks. I told them I had to give some notice to the Wilmington DA," Jane replied.

"That's great! Congratulations," Dan said, as he squeezed her hand.

"So are you going to be okay with me working in the DA's office and you being a Chicago cop?"

Dan smiled. He'd already thought of the possibility.

"I promise I won't abuse our relationship. You can count on that," he answered.

"Let's change the subject."

"Okay. What do you think of Victoria's offer?" Jane asked.

"I think the Conrad home would be a great place to get married. When do you think we should do it?"

"How about a week before I start with the DA's office? That way, we could go somewhere for a honeymoon."

"Sounds great to me," Dan responded. "That means three weekends from this weekend, we get married."

"I guess we're on, then. Should you call Victoria?" Jane asked.

"Let's just go over there. That way, you can see where it would be."

The drive to the Conrad home took 30 minutes. Dan called ahead. Victoria was excited to see Jane again. The last time she'd seen her was in Wilmington, three years before.

"Jane, it's so good to see you," Victoria greeted her at the door.

"Hi, Victoria. It's great to see you."

"James isn't here, but I thought I'd give you a tour of the house and grounds. Is that okay?"

"We're in your hands, Victoria," Dan replied.

For the next hour, Victoria gave them a tour of the Conrad home. She left nothing out. The enormity of the house was evident after the first 30 minutes of the tour. Dan had been to the Conrad home in the past, but he'd never seen it all.

"Victoria, this would be perfect for the wedding. Are you sure you want to do this?" Jane asked.

"Of course I do. It'll be great fun. Besides, we got really close to Dan and Alyssa. It's something we want to do to show how important they are in our lives. When are you thinking of having the wedding?"

"Will three weeks from this Saturday work?"

"It will work just fine, Jane," Victoria responded.

"It's going to be just family and friends. We aren't even sending invitations. Dan and I will contact everybody personally. I would expect anywhere from 30 to 50 people, no more."

"Wait a minute. We'll have more than 100 just from the precinct," Dan injected.

"Dan, what are you..." Jane began.

"Just kidding."

"Sorry, bout that Victoria. Dan has a different sense of humor."

Victoria started to laugh. Soon, all three were laughing.

"It's set, then. Leave everything to me. I'll make sure it's special," Victoria told them.

"I can't thank you enough," Jane said, as she and Dan walked to the front door.

"Dan, I think Alyssa will be here with us on that day," Victoria commented.

"I know. I'm counting on it," Dan replied.

Chapter Forty-Four

Within an hour, Jason had located Silas Thompson, Jr. The Ebenezer Missionary Baptist Church was closed in 1976. The church failed financially due to population shifts. The property had been foreclosed. No buyer surfaced. As years passed, it became an empty shell of what it once had been. The last minister of record was Thompson. He'd moved to Joliet and was now the head pastor at Faith Baptist Church.

"Dan, do you want to go with me to see Thompson?" Jason asked, as he knocked on his boss's office door.

"Yeah, I'll be right there."

Jason waited in the car while Dan finished what he was working on. He had taken Jane back to the house and decided to check in at work.

"Is the Menick report in yet?" Jason asked, as Dan got in the car.

"Yeah - not much help, though. The guy's lived in the same house all his life. His only job was with your grandfather. Nothing unusual. Only interesting thing was that his bank records show a regular $1,000-per-month cash deposit for the last 50 years, and it wasn't salary."

"From who?" Jason asked.

"No way to tell. It was cash."

"When did they start?"

Dan hesitated.

"Around 1952."

Dan gave Jason a rundown on everything he'd found in the Menick background check. Both agreed nothing was suspicious except the regular monthly deposit. The subject changed quickly.

"Jason, do you know Jane and I are getting married at your parents' house three weeks from Saturday?"

"Yeah, my mother called me right after you guys left. I think it's a great idea. Does this serve as my invitation?"

"Yes, yours and Halie's," Dan replied. "So, tell me how you located this guy."

"Actually, it wasn't too hard once I figured out what Internet sites to go to."

"You called Kenny, didn't you?"

"Yes, he found the guy in an hour," Jason admitted.

"Figures. Oh, crap. I need to call and invite them to the wedding."

"They already know about it. Jane called them."

The drive to Joliet during rush hour took more than an hour. Joliet was an industrial city whose industrial base had dried up. The most notable thing about the city now was its prison.

"Joliet. I've put a few guys away here," Dan quipped.

"All I know about the prison is the scene from *The Blues Brothers* where it shows the outside walls," Jason laughed.

"You want to see the prison?"

"No, thanks," Jason replied. "I think we should just head to the church."

They decided to drive by the church to see if Thompson was still there. The church looked surprisingly similar to the old Ebenezer church in Cicero. The primary difference was its setting. Faith Baptist was on a busy, four-lane business street, whereas Ebenezer was in a neighborhood. *After walking through the lifeless Ebenezer, the stark contrast to the apparent vitality of Faith Baptist was sad,* Jason thought to himself. A quick check indicated that everyone had gone home for the night. The building was locked. Jason and Dan proceeded on to Thompson's home.

Silas lived in a middle-class neighborhood not far from the church. The brick, two-story home was small, but well cared for. There were no signs of children. Homes across the street and on each side had children playing in the front yard. Three small children played in a plastic swimming pool next door. The Thompson home stood out. It was clearly a home occupied by adults. The information that Kenny had given Jason indicated that Silas was

58 years old, married to Helen Thompson for the past 35 years, and childless.

Dan rang the doorbell.

"Hello - may I help you?" the middle-aged man said from inside.

"We're with the Chicago Police Department, and we're looking for Silas Thompson," Jason replied.

"My dad died about 15 years ago, but I'm Silas Jr. Will that do?"

"Hello - my name's Jason Conrad, and this is Dan Johnson. We just have a few questions we'd like to ask you, if that would be okay."

"Sure, come on in."

"Reverend Thompson, did you pastor the Ebenezer church in Cicero?" Jason asked.

"Yes and no. I did for about two months. I think you're probably thinking about my father. He served that church from about 1947 till I took over two months before it closed. He lived here with us after my mother died."

Jason looked around the room. On the mantel was a picture of Silas Thompson, Sr., with his wife.

"I'm sorry to hear that," Jason replied.

"That's okay. He lived a good life."

"Are there any church records from Ebenezer?"

"No, they all got destroyed in a fire in 1972. After that, things just went downhill," Silas answered.

"Are there any members from Ebenezer still alive?"

"Oh my, let me think. Lilly Dalton may still be with us. Alice Brown maybe, but she may have died last year. Those are the only two that might still be alive. I wish I could tell you for sure, but I can't. I will tell you they lived in Cicero. I doubt they ever moved."

"Did your father ever mention the name 'Oliver Conrad' to you?" Jason asked.

"No - not to my memory. Is that a relative of yours?"

"Yes, he was my grandfather."

Jason and Dan finished their interview and left. They had two names. They'd hoped for more. They'd hoped for church records and membership lists.

"In the morning I'm going to track down the two names Silas gave us," Jason remarked.

"Good. I'm going to focus on the deposits in Menick's account," Dan replied.

"You'd better get home Dan. You have a fiancée waiting."

"And you don't have someone waiting for you?"

"Good point."

Silas waved goodbye to the two Chicago detectives. As they rounded the corner he walked over to a chest against the wall of the living room. He opened it and pulled out a box of assorted papers and pictures. He sat down on the carpet and laid them out in front of him. He held one up and smiled. It was a picture of his father with Laynie Jessup and a young child. Beside Laynie was Frederick Menick. On the back was a stamped date - March 18, 1951. In front of the child sat a birthday cake with three candles.

"You're secret's safe with me, sweet child," he said aloud to himself.

Chapter Forty-Five

January 1948

"Laynie, where'd you go? I've been worried sick," Oliver said, as Laynie and Frederick entered the back door.

"Oliver, it's my fault. Laynie wanted to talk to her pastor, and I suggested we drive over to see him. I should've known better, but I thought as long as we stayed in the car till we got to the church, it would be okay," Frederick told him.

"No, Frederick. It was my idea, and I take responsibility," Laynie responded. "I needed to get out. I needed the air."

"I thought we agreed that it would be safer if you stayed inside."

"I have to get out sometimes, Oliver. I'm not going to hide. Please understand."

Oliver knew it had to be hard for Laynie. He wanted to walk the streets on sunny days holding her hand. He wanted to take her to nice restaurants and shops. He couldn't. His greatest fear was being seen by friends and colleagues.

"I know it's hard, Laynie, but it's for your safety and the baby's."

Laynie didn't reply. She went to their bedroom and closed the door. Frederick emptied the grocery bags and busied himself cleaning the kitchen. Oliver retreated to his study and a glass of brandy in front of the fireplace. His mind continued to try to come to grips with what he should do.

It didn't take long for Mary Jordan to start spreading gossip. When her husband returned home from work, she asked about Oliver, his driver, and the pregnant colored woman she'd seen. Later that night, she called her neighbor, Lillian Armstrong.

"Lillian, have you ever seen Oliver Conrad's driver?" she asked.

"No, don't believe I have, why?"

"I saw him pick up a pregnant colored woman in front of our house. She sat in the back seat as if he were her driver. Doesn't that seem odd?"

"Yes, it does," Lillian answered. "Who do you think she was?"

"I don't know. I asked Stillwell about it, but he didn't know anything. I'm going to find out what's going on."

Mary Jordan and Lillian Armstrong were the center of Hinsdale gossip. Their network included wives of doctors, lawyers, educators, and businessmen.

"Mary, let's not start spreading rumors, okay?" Stillwell Jordan told his wife, as she got off the phone with Lillian.

"I'm not. I was just asking a friend what she knew. That's all," Mary replied.

"That's how rumors start. You know that."

"Then, why don't you go over there and ask Oliver? Let him tell you the truth. It's the perfect way to stop rumors," Mary responded.

"That would be invading his privacy. Just leave it alone."

Mary turned away and walked into the kitchen. She didn't intend to leave anything alone. She was intent on finding the truth.

Al Savuzzo had removed Oliver and Laynie from his thoughts. His father, Lou, suffering from ill health had given over control of the organization to his son, with some exceptions. A weak heart had taken away Lou's strength. Now it was hard to climb a flight of stairs without getting winded. Where once he worked 18-hour days, now he could barely manage an hour or two at his desk. Most of his time was spent in bed. Sitting at the dining room table, reading the *Chicago Tribune*, Lou was having a good day. His energy was up. His mind was on Oliver Conrad.

"Al, is Oliver Conrad up to date on his account?"

"Yeah, he's current. His tool and die factory closed last month. He just didn't know how to run it. The real estate business has gone real well. He's making plenty of dough."

"I want you to make him rich. I want him to be our front. We find the property. He buys it, with our help, and he takes the risk. Up our cut to 50%, and tell him we still expect our $5,000 a month."

"Okay. Anything else you want me to do?" Al asked.

"Yeah. Keep him close. Whatever it takes."

The Savuzzo family had made Oliver rich. If not for the tips and inside information, the tool and die business failure would have bankrupted him. He was becoming wealthy. His medical practice was expanding. Money was coming in from several sources. He'd gotten used to the affluent lifestyle.

Al asked Oliver to meet him at an Italian restaurant downtown, Genova's. Sitting next to Al was Bruno Caseo. Oliver had yet to arrive. Genova's was a small, dimly lit hang out for the Savuzzo family. A private table at the back of the restaurant was always held for Lou, and now, Al. Red leather booths and black tablecloths made the restaurant even darker. A layer of smoke nested near the ceiling as Al and Bruno puffed on cigars.

"Hey, Al, why are we meeting with Oliver?"

"Just a new deal we're putting in place. We're gonna make Oliver rich, and he's gonna make us richer," Al replied.

"You still trust him? We've had some run-ins with him lately."

"Oh yeah, Oliver's fine. He knows we can make him or break him," Al responded.

Oliver arrived early and joined them at the table. He had an idea that the meeting was about business, but he wasn't sure.

"Hey, Oliver. Sit down - order some lunch," Al directed.

"Thanks, but I ate at the hospital," Oliver replied.

"Too bad, the pasta's great here."

"What did you want to talk to me about?"

"Lou and I are changing our deal with you. We want you to be more active as a front person for us. It's gonna be good for you."

"Good for me - how?"

"Here's the deal. We're gonna give you more leads in the real estate market. You're going to make a killing."

"And what do you want from this?" Oliver asked.

"We give you the leads, help with the funding, and keep you safe. You give us 50% of the profit you make. You take the risk, and we both prosper."

"How about the $5,000 a month I'm giving you?"

Al chuckled.

"That continues. That's sort of like your dues."

Bruno sat quietly, listening. His place was to protect Al - not join in any conversations.

"Do I have a choice in any of this?"

"No, no you don't," Al laughed.

Chapter Forty-Six

Stillwell Jordan didn't like what his wife had become. Her prying nature offended his sense of privacy. Yet, he, too, was curious. Driving to work, he'd seen Laynie in the front yard of Oliver's house. He chose not to tell Mary. He and Oliver were partners in the same practice. Any public scandal would hurt the practice. *It took years to build a reputation and only days to ruin one*, he thought to himself as he walked up the sidewalk to Oliver's house.

Jordan decided to drop in on his partner. It was 7:30 p.m. He knew Oliver was home. He saw his car in the driveway.

"No better time than the dinner hour," he said aloud, as he climbed the steps of the front porch.

Oliver and Laynie had just sat down to dinner. As usual, they were eating in the kitchen. It had become their routine. After dinner, they would sit out on the back porch. Since the confrontation with Al Savuzzo, they'd decided to stay away from the front porch.

"Stillwell, what brings you by?" Oliver asked, as he answered the doorbell.

"Just wanted to talk to you for a minute. Is that alright?"

"Sure, can we talk out on the porch?"

Jordan could see into the kitchen from the front door. Seated with her back to the door was Laynie. It was clear to him that she was eating dinner. Whether Oliver had been with her wasn't clear.

"That would be fine," Jordan replied.

The appearance of Stillwell Jordan at his front door shocked Oliver. It didn't surprise him. He knew Laynie's walk was noticed.

"I'm surprised to see you, Stillwell. Something new happen since I saw you at work?"

Jordan was a senior partner in the practice. Fifteen years older than Oliver, he was one of the founding members of Neurology Partners, Inc. He had to be given due respect - Oliver knew that.

"No, nothing new, just a concern that Mary voiced today that I thought I should clear up before rumors spread. You and I both know she's the center of most of them around here."

"I'd be glad to help," Oliver responded.

Laynie knew Jordan and remembered waving at his wife during her walk to church. She shook her head as she remembered Frederick picking her up in front of the Jordan home.

"I bet he's doing Mary Jordan's bidding," she said to herself as she walked to the front door.

Oliver and Stillwell were engaged in conversation. Laynie listened at the door. Frederick, who heard Jordan arrive, stood at the landing of the second floor. Neither Oliver nor Laynie saw him.

"Oliver, we've been friends a long time, haven't we?"

"Yes, from before medical school," Oliver replied.

"You've been a valuable addition to our practice. I'm glad we added you as an associate. You're up for partnership next year. That would be a substantial bump in your salary," Jordan began.

Oliver knew what was coming. His only surprise was that it hadn't come sooner.

"What's wrong, Stillwell?"

"Please forgive me for asking. It's for the good of the firm. We've spent a lot of time building our reputation and patient base. We can't afford anything that would harm that."

"Stillwell, what is it?" Oliver interrupted.

Jordan looked away. He hated invading someone else's privacy.

"Oliver, do you have a pregnant colored woman living here?"

"Are you talking about my housekeeper, Laynie?" Oliver answered.

"Is she pregnant?"

"Yes. She's due in March."

"Whose baby is it?"

Laynie strained to hear Oliver's response. Frederick watched Laynie. Oliver hesitated before he answered.

"She has a man in her old neighborhood who's the father. I think they're going to get married," he answered.

"Why was your driver driving her around a few days ago? Mary said she was in the back seat as if he were working for her."

"Stillwell, they're friends. She had to go to the store, and he thought it would be better for her to have more space in the back," Oliver replied. "He was just worried about her."

"Well, I'm glad you cleared that up. Now, maybe I can get some peace and quiet from my wife."

"Did you think she was with me and that the baby was mine?" Oliver asked.

"Ah, Mary wondered, but I never gave it a thought."

"Tell Mary that Laynie's the housekeeper. I wouldn't be with my housekeeper. You should know that, Stillwell. Besides, she's colored."

Laynie listened to the discussion. She couldn't believe Oliver's response to Jordan's questions. She sat stunned by what she heard. Oliver denied everything. He denied any relationship existed at all. When put to the test, he opted for safety and his livelihood. Frederick watched from the landing. He, too, had heard Oliver's denial.

Jordan finished his conversation and started walking back toward his home.

"Tell Mary not to worry," Oliver called out.

Jordan waved back.

"Trust me, I will."

Laynie moved back to the kitchen table. Frederick climbed the stairs to his quarters on the third floor.

"He'll never marry me - let alone recognize me and the baby as his before God," she whispered aloud.

"I'm sorry, Laynie. It was a neighbor. You know Dr. Jordan, don't you?" Oliver asked, as he sat down at the table.

"Yes, I do. I know both him and his wife, Mary."

As he and Laynie finished their dinners, both were quiet. Each thought about the meaning of the neighbor's visit. Laynie heard what she feared most - that Oliver wouldn't be able to make their relationship public. Worse yet, he denied being the father of her child. *His admission to Al Savuzzo had been self-serving*, she thought to herself. When it came to his medical colleagues, he couldn't make the commitment.

Laynie excused herself from the table. After washing the dishes, she quickly retired. Oliver left her alone. From her demeanor when he returned from talking to Jordan, he guessed that she'd heard the conversation. Now, he had to deal with the aftermath. Sitting on the front porch, he faced his own weakness.

"You coward. You just couldn't do it, could you?" he said aloud, throwing his brandy glass against the porch wall.

Laynie lay half awake in their bed. She tried to decide what to do. She had seven weeks remaining before the baby was due. It was now clear to her that Oliver Conrad wasn't the man she thought he was. She loved him. She just couldn't trust him.

"I'm going to stay here until you come into this world," she said aloud to her unborn child. "Once you're here, we're leaving."

Chapter Forty-Seven

Frederick sat in his chair on the third floor of the Conrad home, reading a book. It was warm on the third floor, even in the winter. In the summer, the heat became oppressive. Only a ceiling fan made it bearable. Often he wondered how Laynie had tolerated the heat. When he did, he felt weak. He tried to imagine what she must be going through. He couldn't. There weren't any words to express the anguish she had to feel. The man she loved didn't feel her love was worth the risk of his career. *With a baby due in seven weeks, she had to be devastated,* he thought to himself. Although he tried to read, he couldn't concentrate. Every page became a struggle. His mind was focused on Laynie. He wished he could do something.

Laynie fought back tears. What she thought would be a future with Oliver was an illusion. She hated herself for planning her life around him. She knew better. Silas Thompson had told her how difficult Oliver's choice would be. She never doubted Oliver's love - only his strength.

Oliver sat on the porch for hours. Even though the January day was pleasant, the cold air started to be uncomfortable by midnight. Three brandy glasses felt the sting of the porch wall. With each, he scolded his actions. The love he'd professed to Laynie for the last seven months was shallow. He knew it. In five minutes with Stillwell Jordan, he destroyed all that he'd built with Laynie over the past year. As much as he wished he could be different, he knew he didn't have the strength to face public scrutiny.

It was past midnight when Oliver finally left the front porch. He turned off the lights and climbed the stairs to the bedroom. Laynie was already asleep. He pulled a chair up beside the bed and watched her. She looked beautiful, he thought to himself. Her face, innocent and untouched by the lines of decisions made against her heart, showed contentment. He felt compelled to reach out and hold her. He wanted to feel her warmth again. He knew the best time of his life had ended.

"Someday, I'll regret what I've done. Hell, I regret it now, but it's too late," he muttered under his breath.

Crawling under the covers, he reached out to pull Laynie into him. When he did, she pulled away. He didn't force the issue. Slowly, he let go and turned to his side of the bed. He didn't sleep much, thinking about what he'd told Stillwell Jordan. The words reverberated in his mind. He tried to imagine what Laynie must have thought as she heard him deny her existence. The hurt she felt became his constant thought.

Frederick found sleep difficult as well. He wanted to do something to make things better for Laynie. He didn't know how to help. Lying in bed, he felt beads of sweat flow from his forehead. Kicking off the sheets, he felt helpless. He knew he was in love with Laynie, but it didn't matter. He knew she loved Oliver.

It was 2:00 a.m., and Laynie couldn't sleep. Oliver had finally fallen asleep, thanks to the brandy.

"Frederick, are you awake?" Laynie said as she shook him.

"No, no - what's wrong? Are you okay?" he answered.

"Yes, I couldn't sleep. Will you talk to me for a while?"

"Sure," he replied. "Let me get some clothes on."

Laynie moved to the living area and sat on the sofa. Frederick quickly dressed and joined her.

"What's wrong, Laynie?"

"You know. I saw you on the landing," she replied.

"You saw me?"

"Yes, but it's okay. It's actually nice that someone else heard and understands."

Frederick didn't know what to say.

"Won't Oliver miss you?"

"He's sound asleep. Besides, I need to talk," Laynie replied.

"Can I get you something?"

"No, I'm fine. I just want to talk."

It was easy to see that Laynie was upset.

"What're you going to do?" he asked.

"I only know one thing. I'm going to stay here until the baby's born. Then, I'm leaving," she answered.

"Are you sure?"

"Yes, I am. Oliver will never accept us. You know that, Frederick. You heard him tonight. I don't want my baby to grow up around people who can't accept us."

"Where will you go?"

"I don't know, but I can't stay here. I don't want Oliver to ever know where we are."

"Is there any way he can redeem himself?"

"No. It doesn't matter what he says. I don't believe him anymore," she replied.

Laynie moved closer to Frederick. Slowly, as if waiting for him to object, she lifted his arm and placed it around her shoulder. She moved her head into him. He didn't recoil. The cool air of January had finally cooled down the third floor. It felt good to feel the warmth of his body next to her.

"Laynie, what about Oliver?"

"He's asleep. I just need a little warmth, Frederick. Would that be okay?"

Frederick didn't answer. He pulled her into his shoulder and held her.

"Thank you, Frederick."

Holding her close, he could feel the baby kick. It surprised him.

"Put your hand on my stomach," Laynie said, as she guided his hand.

"Oh my, I felt that. Does it ever bother you?"

"No, it's actually comforting. It's nice to know someone depends on you and that you're not alone."

"Laynie, you're not alone. You know that."

"I know, and I love you for being here."

It was 4:00 a.m. when Laynie awakened. Frederick, head back, lay asleep. He hadn't moved since she'd rested her head on his shoulder. Slowly, she lifted his arm from around her and got up. Leaning forward, she kissed him gently on the cheek. Quietly, she went back to her room and crawled back into bed with Oliver.

"Laynie, where'd you go?" he asked.

"I went downstairs for a little while. I couldn't sleep."

"Are you okay?"

Laynie turned away from him. She began to cry as she answered.

"Yes, I'm okay."

Oliver didn't respond. He patted her on the back and fell back to sleep.

Chapter Forty-Eight

August 1952

Miriam and Oliver Conrad had settled into a comfortable, affluent life. Their son James had become the focus of their lives. He was an active, energetic two-year-old. It had been a month since Oliver had given given Lou Savuzzo a lethal dosage of morphine. Living with the knowledge that he had killed someone at Al Savuzzo's behest was difficult. Taking advantage of the opportunity it provided was easy. Unknowingly, Al had held the vial of morphine and the syringe that Oliver had used to give his father the overdose. Now, sitting at his desk, Oliver contemplated how to use what he had. Al was now the unquestioned leader of his family business.

"Oliver, are you okay? You've been in here a long time," Miriam said, after putting James to bed.

"I'm fine. I was just thinking."

Miriam knew her husband. She knew something was on his mind.

"If it's something bad please tell me," Miriam asked.

"It isn't, please don't worry."

As Miriam walked up the stairs to her bedroom, Oliver made his plan. He'd been working on it for the last two weeks. Over those two weeks, he had liquidated more than half of his holdings and had put together a significant cash account. In the morning he would visit Al. In the morning, he would change the direction of his life.

A summer heat wave had hit Chicago, and, even at 8:00 a.m., it was uncomfortable. Oliver decided against calling ahead. Instead, he simply showed up at Al's front door. He knew what he was going to do would be dangerous, but it was the only way.

"Hey, Doc, you're early today," Bruno Caseo remarked.

"Yeah, I know. Is Al here?"

"Sure. I'll get him."

Bruno walked back into the kitchen. Moments later, Al came out.

"Oliver, why are you disturbing my breakfast?"

"I need to talk to you, Al. It's important."

The two men moved into the living room and took seats opposite each other. Oliver felt his hands shaking. Beads of sweat formed on his brow, and he could feel his shirt getting damp. He tried not to look frightened.

"So, what do you want?" Al asked.

"Al, I want out. I want to be left alone."

Al chuckled and looked at Bruno.

"He wants out. Don't you know that nobody gets out?"

"Can you ask Bruno to leave?"

Al motioned for Caseo to leave the room.

"What's so important that you need privacy?"

"I just didn't think you wanted Bruno to know about Lou, did you?"

"No, and remember - it never happened," Al responded.

Oliver reached into his pocket and pulled out a piece of paper.

"What's that?" Al asked.

"This is a list of several items that I've left with a bank. The instructions are to deliver the items to the FBI if anything ever happens to me, my wife, or any member of my family."

Al laughed. "What are you talking about?"

"Remember when you handed me the vial of morphine and syringe when you asked me to end Lou's life? Well, you left fingerprints. I've prepared a sworn statement describing what happened and your involvement. I've also detailed our relationship and everything that's happened over the last seven years."

Al stood up and moved toward Oliver. His face reddened with rage. His fist balled up.

"Go ahead, Al. If you act, be ready to spend the rest of your life in prison," Oliver said, as he rose from his seat. "I've also arranged for a copy of everything to go to all your family members and your church."

"You're dead - so is your wife, son, and everybody in your family," Al screamed in anger.

"You don't want to do that, Al. All I ask is to be left alone. I want out. I don't want you to be involved in my life ever again."

Al sat speechless in his chair. He felt powerless. The fear of the FBI knowing everything was real to him, but worse yet was the thought of his family and church knowing that he'd killed his own father. Oliver approached him and pulled an envelope from his pocket.

"Al, this is a check for one million dollars. This is my buyout. All I ask is that you leave me alone and, that someday, if I need a favor, one favor, it'll be granted."

Al looked at the check and the paper detailing what Oliver had and leaned forward in his chair.

"Oliver, you're out. Consider your account closed. If you ever break your word, I will kill you. You know this," Al responded.

"And the favor?"

"It'll be granted. If not by me, then by Anthony."

"Do I have to worry about what's around every corner?" Oliver asked.

"No - no one will touch you or your family. You have my word."

Bruno Caseo escorted Oliver out of Al's home.

"You got guts," Bruno said, as he opened the door.

"You heard?"

"Yeah. I hear everything that goes on in this house."

"Is his word good?"

"It will be - trust me, it will."

As Oliver pulled out of the driveway, he felt a tremendous sense of relief. For the first time since Lou Savuzzo had approached him in the cemetery after his father's death, he felt in control of his life.

Chapter Forty-Nine

As Oliver drove back to Hinsdale, he thought about how his life felt less complicated and safer. He also thought about Laynie. It had been four years since she'd disappeared. Things had changed dramatically. Now, he was happy with Miriam and James. He still wondered where Laynie was and whether he had another child, but he knew her leaving was the best thing for both of them. He thought about the emptiness he felt when he had come home after a medical meeting in New York to find her gone.

March 1948

The first labor pain came at 7:30 a.m. Oliver had left the day before for a medical meeting in New York City. He hesitated to leave but at Laynie's insistence decided to make the trip. The weeklong meeting would still end a week before the due date. The past six weeks had been difficult for them both. Each realized the relationship would end. Although they still shared a bed, they hadn't touched each other in weeks. Meals had moved to the dining room, and very few included both of them. Neither wanted to talk about the conversation he had, with Stillwell Jordan.

It was springtime, but the chill in the air made it feel like winter was trying to hang on as long as possible. Laynie sat on the back porch, drinking hot tea and reading the *Chicago Tribune.* Frederick sat alone on the third floor, reading a mystery novel. It was quiet and peaceful. The quiet was broken by a panicked call from Laynie.

"Frederick, Frederick!" she called out from the first floor.

Frederick quickly descended the stairs and found Laynie sitting on a chair in the dining room.

"What's wrong, Laynie?"

"My water broke. Can you call the midwife?"

Laynie had found a midwife in the Cicero colored community to deliver her baby. She didn't tell Oliver. She knew he'd object. She wanted no part of a hospital.

"Mrs. Harris?" Frederick asked.

"Yes, the number's in my purse on the kitchen table."

Frederick called Wilma Harris and asked her to come as soon as possible. After hanging up, he helped Laynie upstairs to her bedroom.

"Can you stay with me till she gets here?"

"Sure," he replied as he sat down next to her on the bed. "Let me get a cool washcloth."

For the next 20 minutes, Frederick tried to be a comfort. He replaced the washcloth several times and held her hand during labor pains.

"Let me go check the door. I think I heard the doorbell."

"Okay. Frederick, please don't call Oliver. I don't want him to know."

"You sure?"

"Yes, I'm sure," she answered.

Wilma Harris was standing at the front door. Frederick had never met her. He'd driven Laynie to a meeting place in Cicero to make arrangements but had stayed in the car. A heavy-set woman in her mid-'50s, Wilma walked with a limp but exuded confidence in her demeanor. She'd delivered more than 300 babies in her community and was known for her ability. Using a midwife was a normal form of delivery in the colored neighborhoods in the '50s. Only when complications took place was it considered dangerous.

"Take me to Laynie," Wilma said sternly.

Frederick led her upstairs. It was clear from her apparent animosity that she thought he was the father. Wilma disapproved of interracial relationships, but she wasn't going to turn someone away who needed help.

"Dear me, you're early, girl," she said, as she sat down next to Laynie.

"Mrs. Harris, I'm sorry," Laynie replied.

"Nonsense; we'll get this child out without any problem at all. Tell your man to go boil some water and get plenty of towels," Wilma directed.

Frederick didn't need any direction. Before Wilma had finished her sentence, he was on his way to the kitchen.

"You all seem pretty close. I can tell he cares about you," Wilma said to Laynie.

"Yes, I know. He has a wonderful soul," Laynie replied.

"Is he the father?"

"No, Oliver Conrad is. He owns the house. He's out of town at a medical conference," Laynie replied.

Wilma didn't respond. She was focused on what she had to do. Ten minutes later, Frederick appeared with a stack of towels and a large bowl of hot water.

"Go get more water," Wilma ordered.

Frederick looked at Laynie as he left the room.

"You alright?"

"Yes," she replied. "I'll be fine."

"Get busy," Wilma said again. "Leave the water at the door, and leave us alone. Don't come in here until I call you."

Frederick did as ordered. After putting the additional bowl of hot water outside the door, he pulled a chair out of a neighboring bedroom and sat down to wait. He wasn't going far. Labor for Laynie lasted six hours.

"You're doing fine. It won't be long," Wilma told her as she wiped sweat from her forehead.

"How much longer? I can't take this much longer."

"I think another hour, maybe a little longer. Just keep doing what I tell you. You'll be okay."

Frederick could hear Laynie's moans. He wanted to help but knew there wasn't anything he could do. All that was left was waiting.

Wilma knew something was wrong. She hadn't told Laynie, but she was fairly certain that she was pregnant with twins. She believed it was best not to tell her it might be twins. Thirty years before, Wilma had given birth to twins - one alive, one dead. It took years for her to recover emotionally from the trauma. Where she could feel two distinctive movements of babies two weeks before, now she could feel only one.

"I need to get more towels. I'll be right back," Wilma said to Laynie, as she walked to the door.

Opening the door she motioned Frederick to come closer.

"One of the babies isn't alive. I could feel both two weeks ago, but now I only feel movement from one. I haven't told her. She'll need you when this is over."

Frederick listened intently. It was more than he could grasp.

"Twins - she's having twins? She never said anything about twins," he asked.

"She doesn't know. I didn't tell her," Wilma replied. "I trust you won't, either, no matter what happens today."

A stunned Frederick nodded his head. Wilma closed the door and moved back to Laynie.

Wilma knew what she had to do. As soon as she realized that one of the babies was dead, she administered a dose of Pethidine. She'd used it before to reduce pain during delivery, but more so to cause disorientation in the mother. She didn't want Laynie to recall the events of the delivery. With each passing hour, Laynie became more and more disoriented. She could comprehend well enough to follow directions, but it was clear she didn't understand the full nature of what was going on.

"Push, baby," Wilma whispered in her ear.

Laynie strained to push with everything she had within her. As the head of the first child crowned, it was clear it was the dead baby. Why the baby had died wasn't important. What was important was delivering the healthy baby and, if at all possible, keeping the existence of the dead child secret. Wilma called out to Frederick to come in.

"What can I do?" he asked.

"Just do what I say and don't question me."

The first baby came quickly. Wilma, out of sight of Laynie, wrapped the child in a blanket and handed it to Frederick.

"Go out in the hall and wait for me," she whispered.

"Where's my baby?" Laynie muttered, still under the effects of the Pethidine.

"She's almost here, dear. I need another big push, and we'll be there," WIlma replied.

Laynie pushed and pushed again. The pain was intense as she tried to gather her senses. Frederick had left the room, holding the dead child. He sat in silence, not knowing what to do. Wilma left Laynie's bedside for a moment and walked out into the hallway.

"She's never to know about the dead child - understand?"

"I understand," he replied.

"This never happened. All she needs to know is she has a beautiful baby," Wilma said, as she re-entered the room.

"I see the head, Laynie. She's beautiful," Wilma told her as Laynie gave a final push.

Seconds later, a healthy baby girl lay in her arms. Wilma cut the umbilical cord and swiftly completed what needed to be done. From outside the room, Frederick could hear the crying child. He didn't have a chance to think about life at that moment. He had to deal with death.

Chapter Fifty

Frederick didn't know what to do. In his arms, he held Laynie's dead son. Wilma had left quickly after delivering Laynie's baby girl. The baby was healthy in every respect, and Laynie, though still dazed, was quickly regaining her full senses. The need to act quickly was clear. Whatever Frederick was going to do had to be done before Laynie became aware of anything.

"Frederick, are you out there?" Laynie called out.

Frederick set the dead baby down on the chair and came into the bedroom.

"She's beautiful," he said, as he looked at the baby in her arms.

"She is, isn't she?" Laynie replied.

"What're you going to name her?"

"Sophie, after my grandmother. Do you like the name?"

"Yes, I do. I like it a lot. How do you feel?" Frederick asked.

"I'm a little groggy. Actually, it's all kind of a blur. I'm just glad it's over."

Sophie quickly fell asleep, as did her mother. Frederick needed to act.

He headed to the basement with the dead baby in his arms. He remembered seeing a large trunk under several pieces of furniture covered by blankets and clothing. He laid the body of the lifeless baby boy on a shelf and pulled the trunk out. He pulled the clothing and blankets off the top and saw the name "Oliver Conrad" on a label.

"Fitting that this should be Oliver's son's resting place," he said aloud.

After taking the contents out of the trunk, he went back upstairs. Entering the baby's room, he gathered up several articles of clothing, toys, and a child's blanket. Stopping in the kitchen, he picked up the paper that Laynie had been reading. It was the March 18, 1948 edition of the *Chicago Tribune*. He folded it neatly and tucked it under his arm.

As he sat in the basement looking at the baby, he decided to make the trunk the child's coffin. He couldn't bring himself to bury the child, and he couldn't let anyone know that it had ever existed. *Besides*, he thought to himself, *this way, it will always be close to the family it never would be allowed to join.* He cleaned out the inside of the trunk and laid a blue tarp that he found in the garage on the bottom. Using the baby blanket he had found in the nursery he gently wrapped the body and placed it in the middle of the tarp. On top of the tarp, he placed the toys, clothing, and children's articles. Slowly, he added more blankets, until the trunk was full. Before closing it, he laid out the newspaper, clearly showing the date. It was as if he were etching someone's date of death on a headstone. Once the trunk was full, he closed the top and used a lock he'd found in the kitchen. In order to hide the baby's final resting place, he pushed the trunk back into the far corner and covered it with furniture, tarps, blankets, and clothing.

"I'm sorry," he uttered, as if to apologize.

When he got back upstairs, Laynie was awake. She was nursing Sophie. Her disorientation had passed. She beamed the happiness of a new mother. *What Wilma said was right*, he thought to himself. *No one can ever know.*

"Frederick, come hold Sophie," Laynie said, as Frederick entered the room. "Where have you been?"

"I wanted to give you a chance to rest. You needed it," he replied.

"I'm so glad it's over, but it was worth it," Laynie said, as she looked at Sophie.

"Do you want me to call Oliver?"

"No. I don't want him to know."

"Laynie, he has to know," Frederick exclaimed, as he reached out and took Sophie.

"No, he doesn't. As soon as I can, I'm leaving. I'll be gone when he gets home. Swear to me you'll never tell him about what happened," Laynie pleaded.

"I will if you promise me something," Frederick responded.

"What?"

"That you'll come stay with Rita and my mother."

Laynie had never considered the option. She had planned to return to Alabama and make a home in Birmingham. Her mother's aunt still lived there. She felt like it would be safe - safe from Oliver finding her and from her father.

"Frederick, are you serious?"

"Yes. I've talked to them both. They want you to come live with them. They both said they'd help you take care of Sophie and that they'd protect your secret," Frederick replied. "I knew you wouldn't stay, so I asked them."

"If you mean this, and, if they tell me face to face, then I will," she replied.

Gertrude and Rita came by that same day. Both told her how much they wanted her to move in with them. It wasn't hard to convince her. She had no home to go to. The warmth of the Menick family touched her. The thought of Sophie growing up with so many supportive, loving people around her was comforting.

"Are you sure about this, Mrs. Menick?" Laynie asked.

"Yes, we insist. Rita and I would love to have you and Sophie live with us. Our home's small, but we have room," Gertrude responded.

"How about Frederick? Where will he live?"

"Laynie, Frederick will continue to work for Dr. Conrad. He'll come each Sunday night and stay till Monday mid-day," Rita answered.

Both Gertrude and Frederick nodded in agreement.

"When do you want to move in?" Rita asked.

"I think I'll be strong enough by the day after tomorrow. I want to leave before Oliver returns."

Gertrude smiled.

"Then, we'll look forward to you moving in soon."

Chapter Fifty-One

As Oliver sat in a lecture on Neurology at the annual American Medical Association Convention in New York City, he felt a great sense of relief. The feeling came from not having to face Laynie each day. He knew his relationship with her was over. He didn't know how it would end, but it felt good not to have to face her each day and be reminded of his weakness.

Over the week that he was gone, he'd received several phone calls from Laynie and Frederick. Each time, they reported that everything was normal and that they were going through the usual daily routine. The baby was due in two weeks. As he boarded the flight to return to Chicago, he felt anxious. Helping Laynie get through childbirth and what would come afterward occupied his mind. He had no answers.

"There's no way she can stay at the house," he said quietly to himself. "There's just too much chance of someone coming by."

The flight arrived on schedule. Rain had come into Chicago, and a steady drizzle was forecast to last the entire day. Springtime was unpredictable. The chance of fair skies and high temperatures was just as possible as temperatures in the 30s and snowstorms. Frederick waited curbside.

"Thanks for picking me up," Oliver said as he climbed into the car.

"It's my job, Oliver. How was the trip?"

"It was fine. How's Laynie?"

"I don't know, sir. I spent last night with my mother and came right here this morning to pick you up," Frederick replied.

"Oh, that's right. It's Monday. How are your mother and sister?"

"They're good. Rita still loves her job. My mother loves having her at home."

"Well, how was Laynie yesterday before you left?" Oliver asked.

"She was fine. I think she's ready to have the baby. She's been really quiet this past week. Hasn't talked about much."

The drive from the airport to Hinsdale took 45 minutes. Traffic was slow as rain caused numerous accidents and slowdowns. It was 11:30 a.m. when Oliver walked into the house. Frederick carried the suitcase and trailed behind.

"Laynie," Oliver called out.

Looking around the kitchen things appeared normal.

"Laynie, are you upstairs?" he called out again.

"I'll check upstairs," Frederick said, as he carried Oliver's suitcase up the stairs.

Oliver walked around the first floor, checking each room. He walked out on the front porch and scanned the side yard, but there wasn't any sign of her. Frederick set the suitcase down in the master bedroom and picked up a sealed envelope that had Oliver's name written on it. He knew what was inside. He knew Laynie was gone. The letter explained things.

"Sir, there's no sign of Laynie upstairs. I found this on your bed," Frederick told him, as he handed him the envelope.

"What's this?"

"I don't know, but it has your name on it, and it's in Laynie's handwriting."

Oliver moved to the den and sat down in his favorite chair. He opened the envelope, pulled out a letter, and began to read.

Dearest Oliver,

This is the hardest letter I've ever had to write. I want you to know that I've loved you for a long time. You became the center of my life. I will always treasure our time together, but I have to leave. I know you realize we can never work. I don't want to be a burden for you. You're a wonderful man who deserves the best in life. You will find someone else who will make you happy and who you can live your life with.

Please let me go. I'll be fine. I've gone back to Georgia to have my baby. I have family there. They'll take care of me. I'll write you when the baby comes so you know she's okay. Thank you for loving me. Working for your family and loving you will always bring me warm thoughts. I will treasure the time we had together and the passion and desire we shared. You have so much love to give. Find someone to share that love with.

I'm sorry if I ever brought discomfort to your life. We just weren't meant to be. I will always love you.

Laynie

Oliver dropped the letter on the floor and stared at the unlit fireplace. Laynie was gone. The woman he'd sworn a love to had left. He knew why. It would have happened sooner or later. He'd hurt her deeply. Leaving was her final act of love. She removed from him the burden of ending things.

"Is everything alright, Oliver?" Frederick asked.

"She's gone. She went back to Georgia to have her baby," he replied, handing him the letter.

"I don't understand."

"She heard me talking to Stillwell Jordan six weeks ago. I could tell. She waited until I left on this trip to leave."

"Why?"

"Because she knew I wouldn't have the courage to recognize our relationship and the baby publicly."

"Would you have?" Frederick asked.

"Sadly, no."

"Why not?"

"Because I'm an idiot who lacks the strength to take a chance," Oliver replied.

"I don't understand. You love her, don't you?"

"Yes, but I can't - or I should say won't - take the risk of losing my practice. I've worked too hard."

"I feel sorry for you, Oliver. Laynie's a wonderful person, and she would have made you happy," Frederick responded.

"I know, but it's just too much for me."

Frederick sat down in a chair on the other side of the room.

"Are you going to try to find her?"

"No. I think it would be unfair to her," Oliver answered.

"Maybe that's best," Frederick replied.

As he listened to Oliver talk, Frederick thought about how close he was to his dead son. He was glad he wasn't going to look for Laynie.

"At least he realizes eventually he would hurt her even more deeply," he said aloud to himself.

It had been seven days since Laynie had given birth and seven days since he'd dealt with the death of the twin boy. The smell of death that had existed for several days was gone now. The constant thoughts and dreams of what he'd done stayed in his mind, haunting him. Each time he thought of holding the dead child, he relived the memory.

Chapter Fifty-Two

Present Day

Jackson left messages with Jason, James, and Claire to meet at Jason's house at 9:00 p.m. The results of the DNA tests were in.

"Who was that?" Dan asked, as they drove back to Chicago after meeting with Silas Thompson in Joliet.

"It was a voicemail from Jackson. He ran DNA tests comparing Dad's DNA to the baby's to see if they're related."

"Mind if I come?" Dan asked.

"No - you're part of this now. We'll go straight to the house. I'll take you back to the precinct to get your car after we're done."

By the time they arrived at Jason's, everyone else was standing on the porch, waiting.

"Sorry, guys; we just got back from Joliet," Jason remarked. "I asked Dan to join us."

"Dan, glad you're here," James replied, as he shook his hand.

Each person took a seat at the dining room table. Jackson opened a file lying in front of him.

"I'm sorry it took so long," Jackson started.

"Jackson, cut to the chase. What's the result?" Jason responded.

"James, the baby in the trunk was a Conrad," Jackson said, looking at James.

"Are you sure?" Jason asked.

Jackson paused.

"Yes, 99.5% sure. This baby was Oliver's."

"My brother?" James asked.

"Yes. At least half brother."

The realization that the dead baby was indeed Oliver's took a moment to sink in. Although the evidence had pointed to the possibility, it was still hard to believe.

"Still leaves the question of who the mother was and how it got in Oliver's trunk," Claire stated. "I still think it might have been the housekeeper's."

"I don't understand. How could this happen? How could we not know? He never gave any clue - nothing," James said aloud.

"Are you okay, Dad?" Claire asked.

"I'm alright, but it just seems so unreal."

"We have to pursue the identity of the mother, James," Dan pointed out.

"I know. What did you and Jason find out?"

"We've narrowed things down to three people who know something, but aren't saying anything," Dan related. "Frederick Menick, the driver; Silas Thompson, the son of the pastor of the housekeeper's church; and Al Savuzzo. Everybody else has died."

"We still have to talk to the two ladies Thompson identified," Jason responded.

"That's if they're alive. That's a pretty big if."

"Why not canvass the neighborhood? Maybe there's still someone around who knows something," Claire suggested.

"Good idea, Claire. Why don't you do that while Dan and I follow up on the two ladies Silas Thompson told us about?" Jason asked.

"And me?" James asked.

"Jason told me you talked to Al Savuzzo. Do you think he knows something?" Dan asked.

"Yes - he reacted strangely to my questions about the housekeeper. He knows something."

James felt uncomfortable. The conversation about his relationship with the Savuzzo family was getting too close. At the same time, he knew Al was involved in some way.

"Did you know Bruno Caseo?" Dan asked.

"I met him once - why?" James answered.

"Because he's still alive. He lives in Cicero, not far from Frederick Menick. I talked to a friend at the FBI today. He told me Bruno's living by himself. He's 92 years old."

"Should we talk to him?" Jason asked.

"I think I'd like to go see him with James. Is that okay, James?"

"Are you going to report all of this?" Jason asked.

"No - not till I know more," Dan replied.

The knowledge that his grandfather was the father of the dead baby occupied Jason's mind as he drove to Halie's apartment. She had given him a key. It was late, past midnight, when he finally returned from dropping Dan at the precinct. As he opened the door, he could see the television was on. She'd fallen asleep on the couch while grading papers. He sat down on the floor and watched her sleep. Many nights during their short marriage, he'd watched Alyssa sleep. Halie, like Alyssa, had an innocence that made him want to protect her. He watched her breathe and imagined making love to her. Slowly, he leaned forward and kissed her cheek. Her long red hair draped over her forehead on to her shoulder. As he kissed her, he could smell the scent of vanilla in her hair. He breathed it in.

"Hey, babe, I hope that's you," Halie said, as she began to open her eyes.

"It is. I was just admiring how beautiful you are."

Halie moved forward to invite him on to the couch. Jason lay down behind her and wrapped his arms around her.

"I missed you," he whispered.

"Hold me, babe. You make me feel so safe."

It was 6:30 a.m. when Jason woke up. Halie had showered and dressed.

"I wondered if you were going to wake up," she said, as she kissed him.

"I'm sorry. I must have been really tired. Are you ready for school?"

"Yes. I need to get there early to set up a display."

"Movie night tonight?" Jason asked.

"Sure; you pick the movie. I'll pick the restaurant."

Chapter Fifty-Three

Sitting at his desk, researching the names that Silas Thompson had given him, Jason didn't see Dan walk up behind him.

"Hey, how was last night? Stay with Halie?" Dan asked.

"Dan, don't scare me like that. You just took three years off my life."

"Well, did you?"

"Yes, I did. We fell asleep on the couch."

"She's so good for you. I'm happy for you," Dan smiled.

"Thanks. I wish Jeff could find someone. I talked to him last night. He and Kim broke up. She moved out."

"Jason, are you blind? Jeff's had a thing for Meredith ever since I've known him."

"Yeah, I kinda figured that out a couple weeks ago. He's worried about her. I could tell it was more than just worry. For a long time, I thought it was Claire he liked, but now I know it's Meredith. I think he's in love with her."

Dan pulled up a chair.

"Not to change the subject, but did you find anything on the names Silas gave us?"

"Dead end, literally. Both died within the last five years," Jason said, as he tossed the files on to the desk.

"Too bad."

"I'm still trying to come to terms with the idea that the baby would've been my uncle. I just can't see Oliver involved with the housekeeper. And I for sure can't see him putting a dead baby in his trunk and leaving it there for 60 years."

"Well maybe Claire will find someone in the neighborhood who knows something."

"So, what should we focus on now?" Jason asked.

"I'm going to see Bruno with your dad. I want you to sit on Frederick."

Dan's contact at the FBI had given him the address for Caseo. He asked James to join him because he wanted the opportunity to talk to him alone. James was standing on his front porch when Dan pulled up.

"Hey, James - ready?"

"Sure. Let's go," James replied, as he entered Dan's car.

The trip to Cicero took twenty minutes ordinarily. In rush-hour traffic, it could take up to an hour. Dan had counted on the delay. He needed time to talk. It was 4:45 p.m., and the traffic was heavy.

"James, I know about your relationship with Anthony Savuzzo," Dan said, as they left Hinsdale.

"What are you talking about?"

"I also know you killed Leonard Simpson."

James turned pale. He could feel his heart beat faster. He'd kept his darkest secret from anyone around him. *How could Dan know*? he thought to himself.

"You don't need to deny it. I'm not here to judge you. I'm not going to do anything about it, but it affects this case. I need your honesty."

James hesitated. He looked out the window of the car at other cars passing by. He didn't know how to respond.

"Dan, I don't know what to say."

"Just tell me the truth. It won't go beyond this car."

"Yes, I killed Simpson. I knew if I didn't, you or Jason would. I couldn't let that happen."

"And Anthony?" Dan pressed.

"Anthony's my best friend. He kept me informed of what he was doing for my father. When he found out who was behind the death of Alyssa, he told me. He agreed to take care of Robert Hollis, and I insisted on dealing with Simpson."

"Did Oliver know about your friendship with Anthony?"

"He knew we hung out together in college."

"Have you told Anthony about what we're looking into?"

"No. I told him I wanted to talk to Al about a family mystery, but he didn't press it. He asked me what it was about. I told him I'd tell him when I knew something, so he backed off."

James hesitated to ask his next question for fear of what the answer would be.

"Does Jason know about Oliver's part in finding Alyssa's killers?"

"Yes, he knows about Oliver. He doesn't know about your role. I don't plan to tell him," Dan replied.

Stopping in front of Bruno's apartment building, Dan turned to James.

"We need to talk some more on the way home. Right now, let's see what Bruno knows."

The two-story brick apartment building was no more than a mile from Frederick Menick's house. Dan drove past the building and turned around a block away.

"I'm going to park here. I'd rather not have him see us coming."

According to FBI files, Caseo had worked for the Savuzzo family for more than 60 years. The building he lived in appeared to have been built in the '30s. One of five on the block, it had seen better days. Walking up the street, both men could feel eyes on them. They stood out.

"Let me take the lead here, James."

"Fine with me."

Pulling open the front door, they saw a row of mailboxes with names and apartment numbers written above. Caseo was listed as living in apartment 1B. They turned around and saw the number on the door opposite - 1B. Dan knocked several times before Bruno answered.

"What do you want?" the elderly man said from inside.

"Are you Bruno Caseo?"

"Who wants to know?"

"I'm Dan Johnson, with the Chicago Police Department. I need to talk to you."

Caseo turned the dead bolt lock and opened the door without unhooking the chain lock.

"Show me your ID."

Dan pulled out his badge and held it inside the door for Caseo to examine. Caseo unhooked the chain and pulled the door open. He was bent over and frail looking. His thinning hair was far from the jet-black thick hair he had had as a youth. His clothes were wrinkled and stained. The once-handsome, well-dressed, and powerful man was a shell of what he used to be.

"Damn - aren't you Jimmy Conrad?" Bruno rasped, as he got a glimpse of James.

"Yeah, it's me, Bruno. How you been?"

Caseo had lived in the same apartment for more than 50 years. The apartment smelled musty and stale. It was small and stuffed full of everything Bruno owned. No space went unoccupied. Pull-down blinds purchased in the '60s covered the windows. Stacks of magazines and papers covered the floors. A small television blared the news on a table in front of a recliner. Caseo had never married and had lived alone his entire life.

"Let me turn off the television," Bruno said, as he walked over to the table.

"Thanks," Dan replied.

James looked at the dust-covered pictures on the walls.

"What do you want from me?" Bruno asked. "I don't have much time, so make it quick."

Bruno didn't like visitors. At 92, he appeared both mentally alert and physically healthy, except for a raspy cough.

"Bruno, how long did you work for the Savuzzo family?" Dan asked.

"I don't know the Savuzzos. Who are they?"

"Bruno, we're not here to cause you any problems. Just tell the truth," James remarked.

Caseo gazed out the window at the walls of the building next door. He sighed, as if coming to terms with something that had occupied his mind for years. Suddenly, he began coughing uncontrollably.

"Sorry, I've been under the weather," he said, as he coughed up blood into his handkerchief.

Over the past month, his health had declined. He'd received news from his doctor the day before that he had three to six months of life remaining. Lung cancer was consuming him. Nothing could be done.

"Alright, yeah I worked for them for over 60 years. What of it?"

"Do you remember my father?"

"Yeah, I remember Doc Conrad. I remember you, too. You've been to the house plenty of times."

Dan listened. He had questions he wanted to ask, but it was clear James was on a track that might lead somewhere.

"Yes, I have. What do you remember about my father?"

"I remember the day I blew up his car," Bruno laughed. "I also remember when Lou set him straight on your grandfather's business."

"What do you mean, set him straight?"

"About the fact that his old man's tool and die business was financed by Lou."

James had never heard his father talk about Eli's business. Neither Oliver nor Anthony had ever mentioned the connection between Eli and the Savuzzo family. James knew his father was connected, he just didn't know his grandfather was. It explained how Oliver got involved.

"Bruno, did you ever meet my father's housekeeper?"

Dan listened. He was fascinated by James's line of questions.

"You mean the colored gal?"

"Yes; did you ever meet her?"

"I saw her a couple times, but I never met her," Bruno answered.

"How pregnant was she when you saw her?" James asked.

Before he could catch himself, Bruno answered.

"I'd guess six or seven months."

"You with Al when you saw her?"

"Yeah, we went over to Oliver's house to have a chat. I could see her at the kitchen table. Oliver came out on the porch to talk to us."

"About what?"

"The kid. Damn it - I thought you knew all this."

"Bruno, what did my father say?"

"He said it was his kid. That they were together, if you know what I mean."

Chapter Fifty-Four

Bruno Caseo, clearly seeing his impending death, was open and honest about what he knew. James sensed Dan knew how far to push him and stopped asking questions. He tried to come to grips with the idea that his father was having a relationship with his Black housekeeper.

"How did Al know the housekeeper was pregnant, and why did he care?" Dan asked.

"I'd seen the colored gal out in front of Oliver's house a couple times. I told Al. He told me he needed to see for himself. They thought I was some dumb Italian who didn't know what he was talking about. They were wrong."

"Why are you telling us this now?"

"Cause Al's almost dead, and I've got about six months. I have lung cancer. I need to get some things off my chest. What're they gonna do, kill me?"

Dan looked at James. Both were stunned by what they were hearing.

"Will you talk to the DA?" Dan asked.

Bruno looked down to the floor. He sensed he'd gone too far, yet he felt compelled to keep talking.

"I know someone in the DA's office. I might talk to her."

James couldn't hold back.

"Are you sure my father was involved with the housekeeper?"

"For the last time, yes. He said the kid was his, and they were together, as in a couple."

"What did my father do for Al?"

"Anything he asked. He took a couple of slugs out of my shoulder once. Fixed up any of Al's guys when they got hurt."

"There was more to their relationship, wasn't there?" James continued.

"Yeah. Lou and Al fed him information on real estate. Lou would front the money. Oliver would invest and take the risk. They split the profit."

"How do you know all this?"

"I listened, and I kept my mouth shut. At least until today," Bruno shrugged.

Dan took out a pad of paper and began to take notes.

"Hey, no notes. What I tell you is verbal and just between the three of us," Bruno said, angrily knocking the pad out of Dan's hand.

"Sorry."

"Your dad got rich on his connection to Lou and Al," Bruno said looking at James. "He would've gotten even richer if he hadn't bought his way out."

"What do you mean by bought his way out?" James asked.

"I was with them in 52' when Oliver came to see Al. You were 2 or 3 years old, I think. They asked me to leave the room, but I stayed within earshot. Your dad had proof that Al ordered him to give Lou a shot to kill him. He also had documents he placed in a safe-deposit box, just in case Al went after you."

James hesitated. He tried to grasp what Caseo was telling him. His father had killed someone.

"Went after me?"

"Yeah. Al said he was gonna kill you, your mother, and everyone in your family. It wasn't until he saw what Oliver had and until Oliver gave him a million bucks that he let him out."

"Out?"

"Yeah, out. Out of the business. He asked Al to leave him and his family alone. He also asked for a favor in the future. I don't know if he ever collected on it."

James knew he had.

"Your dad stood up to Al. He had guts," Bruno said as he looked out the window.

"Al let him walk away?" Dan asked.

"What choice did he have? He didn't care about the police knowing he had Lou killed, but the thought of his family and church knowing was unthinkable."

Caseo had watched the inner workings of the Savuzzo family for decades. He had been privy to every event, every action. Both Lou and Al trusted him. Only the need to cleanse himself before he died had brought about this desire to talk.

"Jimmy, you've been involved for a long time. Why don't you walk away like your dad did?"

James felt uncomfortable.

"You don't need to answer. I know you and Tony are close friends. Did you know that Al ordered him to befriend you in college?"

"Befriend me? What are you talking about?"

"Yeah, I heard him tell Tony about you before he went to college. He told him to make you his best friend."

"Why?" James asked.

"I think he wanted to stay close to Oliver. He wanted a little security, just in case."

James had never considered the possibility that the meeting and subsequent friendship with Anthony had been arranged. He didn't want to think that what he had believed to be a true friendship was something entirely different.

"Did you ever see the housekeeper again?" Dan asked.

"Well, let me see. I saw her when she was pregnant a couple times. I also saw her sitting at the kitchen table when Al and I visited Oliver. That's it. I never saw her again after that."

It was easy to see the strain that the visit had caused for Caseo.

"I don't feel well. You guys need to leave."

"Thanks, Bruno. You've helped," James said, as he opened the door to leave.

"Well, at least now I can consider myself even with your dad."

"What?"

"For saving my life 60 years ago."

James stopped before he closed the door.

"Bruno, just one more question."

"One more - then that's it."

"After my dad visited Al in '52, did you ever see him again?"

Bruno chuckled.

"Yeah, one other time. In 1957, he came to Al's house. I saw him there. They met for about an hour. That was the last time I saw him. Funny - Al was white as a ghost when he left."

Chapter Fifty-Five

Dan and James sat in Dan's car without talking. The meeting with Bruno Caseo had changed everything. Questions that were answered brought up new questions that hadn't ever been considered. Dan started the car and turned on the air conditioning. The motor idled as they both looked at Caseo's apartment building. Neither could speak.

"I'm blown away," James muttered.

"Me, too. You know how much information Caseo has stored in his head and most likely on paper in that place?"

"Yeah, I know, 60 years worth. He could put Al and Anthony away for a long time."

"What was that last question about? Why did you want to know when Bruno last saw Oliver?" Dan asked.

James paused. He had an idea, but he didn't want to share it with Dan, at least not yet.

"Just curious, that's all. You know who lives in Cicero, right? Just a few blocks away."

"Yeah, Frederick Menick. Do you think there's a connection?" Dan asked.

"Has to be. It's too big a coincidence. I knew when I talked to him he was hiding something."

Both men looked toward the Caseo building again.

"Do you think Anthony knows anything?" Dan asked.

James tried to recall the visit with Al. Anthony had been present but acted as though he didn't know anything about what he was talking about.

"No, I could tell when I talked to Al that Tony didn't have the foggiest idea what I was talking about. Al sure did react, though. I hit a nerve. I don't know what he was afraid of, but it was something."

"One person holds the key to all of this, James."

James nodded his head. Whatever happened with the housekeeper, Frederick was the link. Now they held the information that might bring the truth from him.

"James, what do think about what Bruno said about your friendship with Anthony?"

As soon as Bruno had mentioned the nature of the friendship, James had begun to think about what it meant.

"I don't know, Dan. It's kind of hard to believe," James replied.

"It is, but I can see it happening. Your father had just spurned the Savuzzos. He had something on them. Getting close to you would be a smart move. If I were Al, I'd have done the same thing. No way Anthony could tell his father no."

"I just can't believe it. We've been through too much together. Makes me wonder if I really know him at all."

"James, it may have been orchestrated, but I think it's a real friendship."

"What about the safe-deposit box Bruno talked about? You think it really exists?" James asked.

"Yeah, I do. It's the only way Oliver could get out. Whatever he had in the box and the money he gave him convinced Al he had no choice," Dan responded.

"How do we find the box?"

"Well, let's start with your memory. Do you remember what banks Oliver dealt with?" Dan asked.

"Only two that I have any knowledge of, First National, and Illinois Bank and Trust. Both are located in Hinsdale. He'd go there every Friday, no matter what."

"Then you'll need to go to each and see if he had a box. I'm surprised it didn't come up at his death. It usually does through probate."

"I don't know, but I'll check tomorrow."

As Dan and James finished their conversation and were about to pull away they saw Bruno exit his apartment building. He walked with a limp and slowly approached the curb. He appeared to be looking for someone. James saw a familiar figure crossing the street two blocks away.

"Stop, don't pull out. Turn off the car," he said to Dan.

"Why?" Dan replied, as he shut down the engine.

"That's Frederick Menick."

Menick met Caseo halfway down the block from Bruno's apartment. They shook hands and embraced. Menick, standing more than six feet tall, made the once-formidable Caseo seem small. A conversation ensued that lasted a few minutes before they walked off together in the opposite direction. As they turned the corner, James and Dan spied Jason's car. He had followed Menick and was observing from a distance.

"Jason, that you watching Menick and Caseo?" Dan asked on his cell phone. "Yeah, where are you?"

"Your dad and I are two blocks up past Caseo's apartment building. We finished talking to him and have been sitting here talking for the last 20 minutes. Caseo must have called Menick after we left."

"What the hell's going on?" Jason asked.

"I don't know, but Caseo told us more than we could imagine. He never mentioned Frederick's name, but it appears they know each other pretty well."

"I've been watching Frederick's house for the last two hours. He came home from the grocery two hours ago and didn't stir. Fifteen minutes ago he shot out of there like a cannon. I could tell something had happened," Jason reported.

"Yeah, I think Bruno called him," Dan replied.

"What do you want me to do?" Jason asked.

"Follow them at a distance. I'm going back in to Bruno's. Let me know if they come back and how much time I have. Don't let them see you."

Dan hung up and turned to James.

"You have my cell. If Jason loses them, and you see them coming back, call me."

James nodded.

Dan exited the car and quickly made his way back to the Caseo apartment. Leaving in a hurry, Bruno hadn't locked the door. Dan didn't need to use the credit card he'd pulled from his pocket. As he walked into the apartment, he was once again struck by the musty odor. Slowly, he walked through each room, surveying what was around him. He didn't want Caseo to know anyone had been there. Starting in the bedroom, he began to lift papers and open drawers. He didn't know what he was looking for. There was no order to anything in the apartment. Personal papers were strewn about in desk drawers, kitchen cabinets, and on top of the dining-room table. In the second drawer of the desk in Bruno's bedroom was a stack of old photos. One of Bruno as a young man next to a pretty, young, auburn-haired woman caught Dan's attention. He turned it over. On the back he read an inscription. "To the love of my life, Rita." Under it was a group photo. As he scanned the photo Dan recognized a younger, fitter Bruno Caseo standing next to an older woman, a young, tall blonde man, and, to his surprise an African-American woman with a child. The child looked to be eight or nine years old. The picture appeared to have been taken at the child's birthday party. A cake with nine candles sat in front of her. On the back of the picture a date, half gone due to age, read March 18, 1957.

Chapter Fifty-Six

Bruno Caseo knew he'd made a mistake. The words had been uttered. He couldn't take them back. The desire to purge himself of guilt before his death had caused him to talk about things long kept secret. At 92, he didn't know when to stop once he'd started to talk. He felt guilty for his misplaced words as he called Frederick Menick.

"Frederick, you need to get over here as soon as you can."

"What's wrong, Bruno?"

"Oliver's boy Jimmy and a Chicago cop just left my place. I talked too much," Bruno replied.

"About what?"

"Laynie."

Frederick felt a chill as he heard Laynie's name.

"I'll be right over."

It took only a few minutes for Frederick to walk to Bruno's apartment. He waited an extra 10 minutes to be sure that Dan and James had cleared out of the area. He didn't see Dan's car. He didn't realize that Jason was following him from a safe distance behind. Bruno met him on the street. They shook hands and embraced. Over the years, they'd become like brothers. The difference in the two men was striking. Although they were within five years of each other, age had taken a far-greater toll on Bruno. Frederick stood tall and erect. His thick blonde hair belied his age. Only a hint of gray could be seen. If not for the deep lines in his face, he could've been mistaken for a man in his 60s. Bruno showed his 92 years. The lung cancer had taken a toll. The ravages of cancer could be seen in his drawn face and withered look.

"Let's take a walk," Frederick suggested.

"Okay," Bruno replied, as they turned the corner.

Neither saw Dan get out of his car and approach the apartment.

"What happened?" Frederick asked as he looked at Bruno.

"I don't know. I just felt like talking. I wanted to come clean. Seeing Jimmy Conrad made me think about the past. He needed to know some things."

"How did Laynie come up?"

"They asked if I ever saw Oliver's housekeeper," Bruno replied.

"Did you mention Sophie?"

"No."

"Thank God."

The secret of Sophie's existence had been kept from the Conrad and Savuzzo families for more than 50 years.

"What're we going to do?"

"Nothing," Frederick replied. "It's too late. Let's not say any more to them, but if they find out the truth, so be it."

"I'm sorry, Frederick."

"That's okay, Bruno. It had to come out some day. Maybe today's the day."

The two old men continued to walk the streets of the neighborhood. It was a neighborhood they knew well. Neither spoke. It wasn't necessary. Frederick thought about Laynie and Sophie. Bruno thought about Rita.

"I'm sorry, too, Bruno. I'm sorry Rita died so young. She loved you."

Bruno Caseo had met Rita Menick at church. He was 35 years old. She was 23. It was 1954. Bruno was the brash, handsome, powerful bodyguard of Al Savuzzo. Although Gertrude warned her not to get involved, she fell in love. Only after Rita had dated Bruno for more than six months did her mother realize what was going on. Frederick had been working for Oliver Conrad for seven years. It had become easy for Rita to slip out at night to meet Bruno. Living only blocks away from each other, their love had grown. Frederick didn't know until a chance meeting at church one Sunday morning. Bruno recognized Frederick as the man he had seen when he glanced inside Oliver Conrad's home and saw him standing on the landing of the second floor. He and Al had come to check on Oliver's pregnant housekeeper.

As he walked beside Frederick, Bruno thought about Rita. It had been more than 50 years since she had died of breast cancer. He remembered how close he'd come to making her his wife. Reluctantly, Gertrude had agreed to the marriage. Frederick didn't believe the news that Bruno had asked his sister to marry him.

"What are you thinking?" Frederick had asked.

"I love him. It's none of your business," Rita had replied.

"He works for a hood. Don't you know that?"

"I know, but he says he's going to quit."

"You don't quit the mob. He'll never get out."

Rita didn't listen. She loved Bruno. No one could dissuade her. The lump she found in her breast changed her future. Three months after their engagement, Rita died of breast cancer. During those three months, she brought Bruno into the family.

"Remember when Rita introduced me to Laynie and Sophie?" Bruno asked.

Frederick chuckled.

"Yes, I don't think I'll ever forget that."

"You thought I'd go to Al, didn't you?"

"I worried you would. Remember, I was at Oliver's when you and Al came over to check on Laynie."

"Yeah, I know. I was a different person back then. Loving Rita changed all that. I would never betray her. This family is now my family," Bruno said

Bruno had never divulged anything to the Savuzzo family. Al never saw the sadness he felt at Rita's death. The funeral, held at the same church they'd met at, was small and private. Only Gertrude and Frederick joined Bruno, Laynie Jessup, and her daughter, Sophie, for the ceremony.

From that moment on, they all agreed that Rita hadn't died but rather moved to New York City.

"I miss Rita every day," Bruno commented. "My life would have been so different if she'd lived."

"Would you really have left Al?"

"In a minute. We would have moved somewhere they could never find us," he answered.

Frederick smiled. He knew how much Rita loved Bruno. He believed they could've been happy together. Bruno had never been with anyone else after Rita. He stayed in the same apartment. His family became Frederick and Gertrude.

"I still don't know how you kept things from Al for so long," Frederick said, as they rounded the corner three blocks from Bruno's apartment.

"Lou and Al were only interested in themselves. They never paid any attention to people like me."

"Dinner Sunday?"

"Sure."

The two men parted a block from Caseo's apartment. Jason called Dan, who had already left the area with James.

"You make it in and out okay?" he asked.

"Yeah, we left. Have they finished?" Dan asked.

"Yes. They're both home by now. Should I stay with Frederick?"

"No, I don't think it's necessary. He's not going anywhere."

Dan thought about the little girl in the picture. He wondered who she was and what her life was like growing up.

Chapter Fifty-Seven

May 1957

Sophie Jessup was nine years old. The death of her aunt six months before had been traumatic. Sophie had never known any family other than the Menicks. Gertrude was like a grandmother, Rita an aunt. The Menicks had adopted Bruno. To Sophie, he was Uncle B. Frederick served as the male role model for the family. Every Sunday, he returned from the Conrad residence and spent 24 hours taking care of what needed to be done. Every Sunday night, Gertrude and Laynie fixed a meal. Laughter and love would embrace the table.

"Let's see, around the table, we have three German immigrants, one Italian of questionable character, and a black woman and her mixed-race child," Frederick laughed.

"I'm glad you waited till Sophie left to say that," Laynie scolded.

"I didn't mean anything bad. I think it's a really good thing. We come from such different backgrounds, yet here we are, together and caring for each other."

"I agree," Bruno responded, looking at Rita

"Here's to you, Rita," Frederick said, lifting his glass. "If not for you, we wouldn't have gotten to know Bruno."

It had been eight years since Oliver had married Miriam. James was now seven years old and would be entering the third grade in the fall. Although she thought about Oliver occasionally, Laynie had moved on with her life. Her daughter was her focus. The non-traditional family that she joined was warm and accepting. Sophie was doing well in the fourth grade at a Cicero public school. Life for Laynie and Sophie was good. Sophie never asked who her father was. She was surrounded by love. She was a typical, well-adjusted, happy adolescent. Her days were filled with school. She was an achiever, always making A's and pleasing her teachers. Quick to make friends, she excelled at attracting children her age. If no one was available to play with she made up games and recruited her mother, Frederick, or Bruno. As a mixed-race child, she was lighter skinned then Laynie. She noticed the difference but never asked her mother about it. Since moving in with the Menicks, Laynie hadn't ventured out of Cicero. Everything she and Sophie needed was provided.

Sitting at the dinner table after Sophie had left to do her homework, Laynie looked at Bruno.

"Bruno, why do you stay with Al?" she asked. "He's an evil man."

"I've worked for him and his father for 15 years. I don't know what else I could do. I used to be a lot like him until I met Rita and this family. If I can keep you all safe by staying close, I will."

Laynie listened quietly, rubbing her forehead.

"He's right, Laynie. We can trust Bruno," Frederick responded.

"Will you excuse me?" Laynie asked.

"Are you okay?"

"Just a headache," Laynie replied.

Frederick followed her back to her bedroom, out of hearing range of Sophie.

"Laynie, is it happening again?"

"Yes, just help me get to bed."

Frederick wasn't worried about Al Savuzzo. His concern was for Laynie. Over the past three weeks, she'd suffered debilitating migraine headaches. Bouts of dizziness meant days spent in bed. Being stoic, Laynie never complained. The week before, she had fallen coming off the front porch steps. Thankfully, Frederick was there. Carrying her back inside, he laid her on her bed.

"Laynie, we need to get you to a hospital. Something's wrong."

"No, I don't want to go to a hospital," Laynie replied.

"Why? You're getting worse. You've had a headache for three

weeks, and your equilibrium is getting worse."

"No. I'll be okay," she responded, as she drifted to sleep.

It was Tuesday, the second day of school for Sophie. Frederick, who had returned to the Conrad residence the previous day, woke early and sat at the kitchen table, waiting for Oliver. As usual, Oliver was timely. James would be waking in an hour to get ready for school. Miriam would rise 15 minutes before James.

"Frederick, what are you up to this beautiful fall morning in Chicago?"

It was a beautiful day. Temperatures were expected to be in the 70s under fair skies.

"I need to talk to you, Oliver."

"Why so glum? What's wrong?"

"I need to tell you something, and I need you to let me finish without interruption. Is that okay?"

"Sure. I hope it's not bad news."

"No, but I want you to know I did what I did because I thought it was best for everyone involved."

For the next 20 minutes, Frederick told Oliver about Laynie and Sophie. He left nothing out, except for the presence of the baby's body in the trunk in the basement. Oliver sat in silence, trying to grasp what he was hearing.

"We need your help, Oliver," Frederick stated.

Oliver stared at the wall, unable to respond.

"Laynie's been staying at your mother's house this whole time?"

Frederick paused to gather his words.

"Yes. She's part of our family now. So is Sophie."

"Sophie. My daughter? Are they okay?"

"Yes. Sophie's nine and in the fourth grade. She's a very smart young lady."

"And Laynie?"

Staring out the window, Oliver thought back to happier days, when Laynie had been the center of his life. He knew when she left that it was for the best. He knew he couldn't find the courage to make their relationship public. Now he had Miriam and James. They were the center of the world for him.

"Does she hate me?"

"No Oliver. She forgave you long ago. Her life now is about Sophie. That's why I'm here."

"What do you mean?"

"We need your help," Frederick responded. "Laynie's ill. Something's wrong with her."

"What's wrong?"

"Over the last three weeks, she's been having severe headaches, nausea, and dizziness. She's spent days in bed. I've tried to get her to go to the hospital, but she refuses."

"What can I do? Will she see me?"

"We want you to come look at her. You're the only person we think she'll talk to or open up to."

"We?"

"Gertrude, Bruno, Rita, and me."

"Bruno?"

"Yes, he is engaged to my sister Rita. He's like family now."

"The same Bruno who works for Al?" Oliver asked.

"Yes."

"Wow, Bruno Caseo, Al's bodyguard. This is all too hard to believe. Wait a minute - I thought Rita moved to New York."

"No, she lives with us here in Chicago."

"How did she meet Bruno?"

"At church."

Frederick knew Miriam would be coming downstairs at any minute. He needed to draw things to a close.

"Will you come over tonight and see Laynie?" Frederick asked.

"Yes, I will, but I can't promise anything."

Chapter Fifty-Eight

The day dragged by for Oliver. He was unfocused and had to postpone his afternoon surgery schedule. Thoughts of Laynie and the past nine years occupied his mind.

"How could they have kept this a secret for so long?" he said aloud to himself sitting at his office desk.

For the past nine years, Frederick had taken off every Sunday afternoon and returned on Monday. During those 24 hours, he'd established a different life. He never mixed the two. While at Oliver's, he did everything possible to support the Conrad family. Although quiet and reserved, Oliver and Miriam knew they could count on him.

"Hi, Miriam. I'm going to be late tonight. I have a meeting I have to attend, so don't wait up."

"Okay Oliver. Is everything alright?"

"Yes, it's fine. Tell James I'll see him in the morning."

James Conrad was seven years old. As an only child, he was expected to do well. Oliver had established a plan for him. He would follow in his father's footsteps and become a physician. The best schools would prepare him for his career and his life. Oliver had become hardened through his experiences. Discipline and appropriate behavior was something James learned at an early age. Miriam provided the soft side to the family. Her gentle, loving way gave him emotional strength. Miriam, unlike Oliver, chose to look for the good in people. When Oliver met her, she was working three jobs in order to help support her family.

Miriam Sample grew up having to struggle for the simple things in life. Coming from a blue-collar family, she had to work for everything. She was 19 when Oliver met her. Her long blonde hair and blue eyes made an impression on the young Conrad. He hadn't seen anyone since Laynie had disappeared. He had reconciled himself to being alone. He wasn't looking for a relationship. Asking Miriam on a date was the result of a dare from a friend. Falling in love didn't take long. By their fourth date, he knew she would someday become his wife.

Miriam had a calming effect on him. Being with her seemed right. Seven months later, they were married in a small wedding at the Fourth Presbyterian Church in Chicago. They honeymooned at Niagara Falls. The first time they made love was on their wedding night.

"I love you, Oliver," Miriam whispered as she lay in his arms.

"I love you, too," Oliver replied, kissing her.

The birth of James 11 months later was a joyous event. Due to complications in the delivery, Miriam couldn't bear any more children. James would be the center of the Conrad family.

Oliver never shared anything with Miriam about Laynie Jessup. He and Frederick had an unspoken agreement to move forward with life and not look back. They didn't talk about Laynie or what had happened. The idea that he might have another child in the world had entered his mind on numerous occasions, but he had been able to put the thought aside. When Laynie disappeared, he made inquiries about her whereabouts but shortly thereafter abandoned the search.

Life was good for the Conrads. It had been five years since Oliver had broken away from Al Savuzzo. During those years, he'd worked hard in his medical practice and in his real estate business. He'd built up a significant fortune. He focused on his career, Miriam on raising James. Even without the tips from the Savuzzo family, he made wise decisions and purchased property at the right time. He was becoming known in Chicago for being as good at real estate as he was at surgery.

At 5:00 p.m. he closed his office door and headed to the parking garage. He'd spent the last three hours of the day trying to think of what could be wrong with Laynie. He tried to imagine what it would be like to see her again. Knowing that he had failed her ate at him. Getting her better now would be the only way he could atone for his weakness.

"I can't believe I've never been to Frederick's house before," he scolded himself.

The directions he'd been given took him by Bruno Caseo's apartment. Nothing in Cicero looked familiar. Not until he drove by Ebenezer Baptist Church did he realize where he was. He remembered the day he had gone to church with Laynie. It had been their first venture away from home, and his discomfort in the environment had been apparent. He thought about how she tried to make him feel at home. It was at that moment that he knew he didn't have the courage to make their relationship public.

As he approached the Menick home, he slowed down. Stopping a block away, he sat in his idling car, thinking. He took a minute to look around. It was a pretty day. His heart rate increased as he turned off the engine and started walking toward the house. At one point, feeling dizzy, he stopped and leaned against a street lamp.

Laynie Jessup was equally nervous about seeing Oliver. Hearing him deny her existence to Stillwell Jordan had hurt her. Yet she understood. Forgiving him was easy. Frederick had told her of Oliver's impending visit only a few hours before he was to arrive.

"Laynie, don't get mad, but Oliver's coming over. I told him everything. He agreed to come see you. If you won't go to a hospital, then maybe he can help."

Lying in bed, she didn't object. The headaches had gotten progressively worse.

"Okay. This is killing me, Frederick."

"I know. You need help."

Laynie had no time for self-pity and recrimination. Her focus was on providing a life for Sophie. The Menicks had welcomed her with open arms. They'd made her part of the family. The death of Rita had tested them. Gertrude's strength had held the family together. They mourned Rita's death and welcomed Bruno into their midst. They were tight knit and protective.

Frederick never told her about the baby who had died. She had no recollection of the events of that day. The midwife had since died, and only Frederick knew the truth. The knowledge that one of her twins had died would have devastated her emotionally. Frederick would not let that happen. Oliver rarely, if ever, ventured into the basement, and the trunk was securely stowed in a dark corner.

Oliver rang the doorbell. From inside, he could hear a child's voice.

"I'll get it," Sophie called out. "May I help you?"

Oliver stood frozen. He couldn't reply. His focus was on the child standing before him.

"Oliver, Oliver, come in," Frederick responded.

Chapter Fifty-Nine

Present Day

Jason looked at a blank piece of paper on his desk. The events of the past 36 hours kept repeating themselves in his mind. He still couldn't believe the revelations about his grandfather. It wasn't the grandfather that he had known.

"Hey, Dan, what do you think is going on between Bruno and Frederick?" he asked, as he opened Dan's office door.

"Got me, Jason, but I'm guessing it involves the housekeeper. We need Frederick to open up. I don't think we'll get any more from Bruno."

"Why do you think Bruno opened up to you?" Jason asked.

"He says because he's dying. He has only a few months to live."

"Is he willing to go to the DA?"

"I don't know. He said he knows somebody in the DA's office. That's hard to believe, knowing who he worked for," Dan replied.

"What did my dad think of your interview?" Jason asked.

"We're both still trying to figure it out. I didn't tell him, but I saw two pictures in Bruno's house that we need to consider. One was of a young woman with a message written on the back. I think she was Bruno's girlfriend. The other was a group shot at a birthday party for a little girl. I could recognize Bruno, Frederick, and I believe Frederick's mother. The other adult was a Black woman. I think she was the housekeeper, and my bet is the little girl was her daughter."

Jason sat across from Dan, listening intently.

"Why do you say that?"

"Because the birthday cake had nine candles and the date on the back of the photo was March 18, 1957. That means she would have been the same age as the newspaper in the trunk. Do you think that's coincidence?"

"Not hardly," Jason replied.

"Me, neither, but it kind of shoots a hole in the theory that the dead baby was the housekeeper's."

"What if she had had twins, one lived and one died? The dead baby ends up in the trunk, and the live baby turns into the young child you saw in the picture," Jason conjectured.

Up to that point, Dan, Jason, and everyone else had assumed the dead child was the only child involved. It was Oliver's. The DNA had proven it.

"Possible, I guess. You know what that means?" Dan remarked.

"Yeah, I have an aunt out there that I've never met."

"Yes, and James has a half-sister," Dan replied.

"What do we do?"

"We go back and talk to Frederick."

It was 2:30 p.m., and Jane was expected in soon from Wilmington.

"We need to make this quick, okay?" Dan commented.

"We will."

The drive took 15 minutes. Dan parked around the corner, not wanting Frederick to see him coming. Frederick sat on the front porch. He waved as Dan and Jason walked up the sidewalk.

"What brings you back, Jason?"

"Hi, Frederick, this is Dan Johnson, my supervisor at Precinct 71."

"Mr. Johnson, glad to meet you. Jason, take a seat; I'll get another chair."

"That's okay, Mr. Menick, I'll just lean on the railing," Dan responded.

Jason took a seat next to Frederick. It was mid-afternoon. A cool breeze was blowing off Lake Michigan.

"Mr. Menick, I'll be direct. We need some answers. I believe you have them," Dan started.

"What are you talking about?"

"Do you know Bruno Caseo?"

"No, don't believe I do," he replied.

Dan looked at Jason and then back at Frederick.

"That's a lie. We both know it. We talked to Bruno a few days ago. We saw you meet with him. You were engaged in a pretty lengthy conversation."

"Okay, I know Bruno. So what?"

"How do you know him?" Dan asked.

"He was once engaged to my sister, Rita. She died before they got married."

Dan now knew who the pretty, auburn-haired woman in the picture was.

"You knew he was Al Savuzzo's bodyguard?" Jason asked.

"Yes, but only after Rita had already gotten involved."

"What happened to Rita?" Dan asked.

"She died of breast cancer in 1958."

Jason sat spellbound by the unraveling connections that existed around his grandfather.

"You were working for Oliver Conrad at that time?"

"Yes sir. I retired four years ago, when he died."

"Mr. Menick, when I was in Bruno Caseo's apartment, I ran across a picture taken at a child's birthday party in March 1957. You were in that picture, as was Bruno. Do you remember the party?"

"No, I don't. Sorry, but I can't help," Frederick replied.

"Was your mother in the picture?"

"Probably, if it was taken here. She lived here until 1982."

"Two other people were in the picture - a Black woman who looked to be in her late 30s or early 40s, and a child. Who were they?"

"I don't know what you're talking about, Mr. Johnson. I'd appreciate it if you both would leave. I'm tired. Unless I'm under arrest, I'd like you to go," Frederick responded, clearly upset by the line of questions.

"Alright, but, I assure you, we'll be back. We want the truth," Dan replied.

As they walked back to their car, Jason wondered why Dan hadn't asked about the dead baby in the trunk.

"I know what you're thinking. I'm holding that back for the right time. Don't worry - it'll be soon."

"Okay, just wondered," Jason replied.

Neither spoke on the drive back to the Precinct.

"Dan, this is getting bigger than I imagined it would. How long can we keep it under wraps?"

"Not much longer, I'm afraid. More and more people are coming into this. The connection to Oliver, the Savuzzo role - it's just getting too big. I'm surprised the FBI hasn't shut us down."

Chapter Sixty

Shift change was in progress at the Precinct when Dan and Jason got back. They agreed to meet in the morning and discuss what they would do next.

"I'm calling it a day," Dan told Jason, as he headed out of the Precinct.

"Jane coming in today?"

"How'd you guess?"

"You wore a tie. Are you picking her up at the airport?"

"Yes. You know Saturday's the big day," Dan laughed.

"We all know that, Dan. I'll be there. So will Halie."

"How're you guys doing?"

"We're great. Never better," Jason replied.

Jason and Halie were now living together. Only daily trips to check his mail took him back to the Conrad mansion. The school year had ended. Halie focused her attention on the new relationship and preparing for the next school year. With her lease nearing renewal the subject of living arrangements had come up.

"Why don't we move to my place? You don't need this apartment. You can save a lot of money. You've been to the house. It's huge. It needs you there," Jason told her.

Halie laughed and kissed him.

"What's your hesitancy?" he asked.

"I don't know. Maybe I'm afraid you're going to dump me. I'd have nowhere to go."

"First, I'm not going to dump you. You're more likely to dump my sorry ass. And second, I'm in love with you. I want you with me in the house."

"Okay, but do I have to clean the entire place? It's huge," Halie replied.

"No, I'll hire a cleaning service. I don't want you spending your time cleaning when you could be making love to me," Jason responded.

Halie laughed. Over the weeks, their relationship had grown. The comfort level was now there. Small inside jokes made them laugh together. Just looking at each other made them smile.

"When do you want to do it? Your lease is up next week. How about I get Jeff, and we move you Friday? I'll take a day off," Jason suggested.

"Okay, but remember - we have a wedding to go to on Saturday."

"As if I could forget that. Dan reminds me daily."

"Did I hear that you're his best man?" Halie asked.

"Yes, he twisted my arm."

"That's great. I'm glad for him. He seems really happy."

"Yeah, he's ecstatic. I have to try to keep him grounded," Jason laughed.

Without hesitation, Halie crawled on top of Jason on the couch and kissed him.

"You know how much I love you?"

"Yes babe - just as much as I love you," he answered.

It had been two weeks since Dan had seen Jane. During that time, she'd given notice in Wilmington and had prepared to move. Her start date with the Chicago DA was in two weeks. A honeymoon with Dan to St. Bart's would follow the wedding. Over the past week, she'd had several conversations with Lisbeth Williams, her new boss. Williams was a workaholic who prided herself on her conviction rate. As the first African-American senior ADA, she put pressure on herself to outperform her fellow ADAs. Jane knew she was in for long hours and an intense environment.

Dan waited in baggage claim for her to arrive. She'd hired a moving company to move her belongings but carried two suitcases full of clothes.

"Hey, sweetheart, you're a sight for sore eyes," Dan remarked as he hugged her at the bottom of the escalator.

"Oh, Dan. It's been a long week. The move was more than I anticipated. Most of the stuff I put in storage until we can look at it together, but there's still quite a bit that's coming up. I hope you have some room."

"Don't worry. We have plenty of room," he laughed.

"God, I love you," Jane said, as she kissed him.

Dan grabbed the suitcases and led her to the car.

"See, we even have a nice day for you. That's pretty rare in Chicago. You're gonna have to get used to the weather."

"I have a lot to get used to. Lisbeth Williams may be harder than the weather."

"She can't be all that bad, can she?" Dan asked.

"No, she's just extremely focused on her job. More so than anyone I've ever known. It's like she has this passion to put criminals away."

"Well that's a good thing, right?"

"Yes, and no. Sure will make for some long days and nights. I hope you're ready," Jane commented.

"I'll be fine as long as you're next to me in bed each night."

The drive to Dan's house took 30 minutes. He'd moved most of Alyssa's things to the basement in preparation.

"Do you and Jason still go to the cemetery?" Jane asked, as they drove past the entrance.

"Oh yeah. Sometimes Halie comes."

"Speaking of Halie, how're they doing?"

"I wouldn't be surprised if Jason asks her to marry him. He's in love. I can see it in his eyes. Last time I saw that look was when he was with Alyssa."

Jane knew it had to be hard for Dan to watch Jason with another woman. The love that was once for Alyssa was now for someone else.

"Are you okay with that?" Jane asked.

"I'm fine with it. Alyssa would be pleased. Halie's a wonderful girl.

Jason will be lucky to have her."

Jane reached out and squeezed his hand. As Dan pulled the car into the driveway she looked around her new neighborhood. Walking up to the front door, Dan turned and embraced her.

"Welcome home, baby," he said, as he swept her into his arms and carried her through the front door.

Chapter Sixty-One

The conversation with Bruno had spurred James's interest in finding out the truth. Now that he knew that Oliver had fathered a child with his housekeeper, his desire to solve the mystery had intensified. He knew the best way to help would be to find the safe-deposit box.

He checked first with the two banks that he knew his father used. Neither had a safe-deposit box in his name. Thinking logically, he proceeded to check every bank in the city of Hinsdale. Again he ended up empty handed. Being a physician, he decided to approach the task in a scientific manner. Over a three-day period, he mapped out on a grid every bank within a three-mile circumference of Hinsdale. The list included both large and small banks.

"How's the search going for the safe-deposit box?" Jason asked his father, as he entered the house.

"Hi, Jason. Slowly, I'm afraid – but I'm not giving up. I know it's out there somewhere."

"How are you doing the search?"

James showed him the list of banks within the three-mile area and the results of his calls.

"I'm going to expand it mile by mile till I get a hit."

"Sounds like a pretty logical approach," Jason responded.

"Frankly, I don't know any other way."

"You remember Kenny Conrow? You mind if I give him a call and see if he has any luck? He's amazing on the computer."

"Sure, go ahead. He should be graduating soon, shouldn't he?" James asked.

"Yes, and I'm glad you brought that up. I promised Kenny and Melinda that I'd check into possible residencies in the Chicago area. I told them you'd be a good connection."

"I'd be glad to help. I know most of the Residency Directors in the good programs. What are they looking at?"

"Melinda wants Orthopedic Surgery, and Kenny's focused on Cardiology."

"Let me call Vince Lee over at Northwestern. He runs the Cardiology program, and Linda Shannon at Cook County has a really good Ortho program. Are they good students?"

"The best. They also have great board scores. Kenny actually graduated number one in his class and was in the 99th percentile on the boards."

"Okay. I'll set them up for an interview."

"Thanks, Dad. I'll call Kenny."

The search for the identity of the baby had given James a sense of purpose that he'd lost. He knew he would never practice medicine again, but he decided he would do whatever he could to help others reach their goal. Helping Kenny and Melinda seemed natural. On his drive to the Precinct, Jason called Kenny.

"Kenny. How you doing?"

"Hi, Jason. We're just getting ready to go to our rotations. We're in Wilmington this month. Melinda's doing a Surgery rotation, and I'm in an Ortho elective."

"Well, I have a couple things I need to talk to you about. First, are you getting nervous about the wedding?"

"You mean Dan's?"

"No, I meant yours, but you're coming to Dan and Jane's wedding, right?" Jason asked.

"Yeah, we're flying in on Thursday night. Can you pick us up?"

"Sure, and you're staying with Halie and me at the house."

"We can't wait to meet her. So she's moving in with you. Sounds pretty serious."

Jason smiled. He knew how serious it was.

"It is. She's great. You'll love her."

"Can we all get together Friday night?" Kenny asked.

"Oh yeah. We're having a party at my house. I've got Claire and Jackson, you and Melinda, Halie and me, Jeff Dodson and whoever he brings, Dan and Jane, and a couple other friends I think you'll like coming. Hell, even Meredith and her mystery man are coming."

"Mystery man - what do you mean?"

"She's dating this guy no one knows anything about. I think she's in love. It's too bad, because I think Jeff's in love with her."

"Jeff? You're kidding."

"No, he told me a couple weeks ago. He wants to check the guy out so Meredith doesn't get hurt."

In the background, Jason could hear Melinda telling Kenny to hurry up. They had to get to the hospital.

"I hear Melinda, Kenny, so I'll wrap this up quickly. My dad's setting up interviews for her at Cook County and you at Northwestern. I'll let you know when. Are there any times you can't come?"

"Hell, no. Whenever he gets it set, we'll be there."

"One other thing. Can you do me a favor?"

Kenny laughed. He knew what was coming.

"Let me guess. You need my computer skills?"

"Yes. We're trying to locate a safe-deposit box in the Chicago area in my grandfather's name."

"You mean Oliver?"

"Yes. It would be at a bank within, I would guess, a 30-mile radius. It might be a big bank, but, more than likely, it's at a small bank."

"How long ago did he take it out?" Kenny asked.

"Probably between 1950 and 1960, give or take a couple of years."

Kenny hesitated.

"I'll try, but, back then, things were done by hand."

"Just give it a shot," Jason replied. "Let me know if you find anything, and tell Melinda about the interviews. I'll see you at the airport on Thursday. Three o'clock on Delta, right?"

"You got it. See you Thursday."

Chapter Sixty-Two

It was Thursday. Only two days remained until the wedding. Victoria had made all the arrangements. Jane's new boss, Lisbeth Williams, would be in attendance. More than 70 of Dan and Jane's family and friends would be there.

"Are you sure Victoria's okay with 70 guests?" Jane asked.

"Yes, I talked to her yesterday. She said she has everything set for 80. Don't worry. It will all be fine."

"I'm just a little nervous," Jane laughed.

"So am I, but it'll be okay."

"Has your family arrived?"

Dan paused.

"They all come in tomorrow. I think they'll love you, sweetheart."

"You have a much bigger family than I do. Only my sister and brother-in-law will be here," Jane replied.

"I'm working only half a day today. I have a meeting with Jason at eight, but how about we meet for lunch and spend the afternoon together?"

"That sounds like fun. Are we going to Jason's party tonight?" Jane asked.

"Oh, yeah. Wouldn't want to miss that," Dan replied.

Dan had kept everything about the baby's remains secret. It had been more than three weeks. Time was running out. He looked forward to the wedding and honeymoon, but he knew it would slow things down.

"Hey, Jason," Dan said, as Jason entered his office for the 8:00 a.m. meeting.

"Hi, Dan. Getting nervous yet?"

"No, not yet. Looking forward to your party, though. Who all's coming?"

"Everybody - all my siblings, friends from here, Wilmington, and a few others. It should be a blast. I'm picking Kenny and Melinda up this afternoon."

"Has James had any luck finding the safe-deposit box? That's what we're meeting about, right?"

"No, he hasn't, but he's going about it in a systematic way. He'll find it," Jason replied.

"You know somebody has to be paying the fees on that box. Otherwise, the bank would report it as abandoned property. The state would take the contents."

"Could Oliver had prepaid the box for years in advance?"

"He could have, but it's been a good while."

Jason hesitated to tell Dan about asking Kenny to search for the box, but he knew he would eventually guess.

"Okay, I gotta tell you. I asked Kenny to see if he can find the box."

"Jason, I expected that. That's not news. Any word yet?"

"No, he's still trying to find information on the housekeeper as well."

"What we need is to find the housekeeper. She would be about 90 years old now," Dan commented. "Maybe we should focus on finding the little girl. She'd be a little older than your dad."

"Yeah, that's the hard part."

"Well, we have three big sources of information still out there. We have Frederick, the safe-deposit box, and Bruno."

"Don't forget the $1,000-a-month deposit in Frederick's account and Silas Thompson, Jr.," Jason added.

"Silas - why Silas?"

"I think he knew something."

"You didn't say that when we talked to him," Dan pointed out.

"I know, but the more I've thought about the meeting, the more I think he's hiding something."

"What?"

"I think he knew the housekeeper or maybe her daughter."

"Let's change the subject for a second," Dan replied. "Do you know, and I want this not to leave this room, that the Chicago DA's office is about to indict Anthony Savuzzo on extortion charges?"

"Anthony? When?"

"I think he'll be arrested today. Apparently, several merchants have come forward claiming he was extorting money from them for personal security services that didn't exist."

"Does my dad know?"

"No one knows. You can't tell him."

"How did you find out?"

"Jane told me Lisbeth Williams has targeted Anthony and his cohorts. Apparently, she's decided to go after him," Dan replied.

"Do you think Bruno had anything to do with this?"

"I don't know."

The idea that the Chicago DA had talked to Bruno and that his information could be the source of why indictments had been issued gave both Dan and Jason cause for concern. Bruno was close to Frederick. The connecting lines led to the housekeeper, the infant, and, finally, to Oliver. As of yet, James didn't know that his half-sister could be alive somewhere.

"What do we do?" Jason asked.

"Nothing. We wait. We continue to press for more information until we're told to back off. Press Kenny for what we need."

"I'll try, but I don't know if he can find it."

"Just keep pushing."

Jason and Dan spent the rest of the morning pursuing leads. They left together. Dan needed to meet Jane. Jason had promised to pick up Kenny and Melinda. Traffic was heavy and the weather dreary. Low-hanging clouds had blocked the sun all morning.

"I hope they get in on time," Jason commented.

"Me, too. I hope they like me," Halie replied.

"They'll love you. Kenny's a computer nut. He's a great guy, but very intellectual. Melinda's a beauty queen. They're total opposites. Melinda comes from a wealthy New England family. Kenny's dad works at a grocery in the mountains of North Carolina. It's fun to watch them because it's clear they're in love. As different as they are, it really works."

"They sound like a fun couple."

"Well, if they get the residencies they want, we'll probably see a lot more of them. They want to come to Chicago."

As Jason finished his sentence, they pulled up in front of the arriving terminal. To their surprise, Kenny and Melinda were waiting curbside.

"What the heck. You guys are early," Jason said, hugging Melinda.

"We caught an earlier flight that got us here about an hour ago," Kenny replied.

"Why didn't you call?"

"We didn't want to bother you. We both had a lot of studying to do," Melinda responded.

They climbed into the back seat of Jason's car. Halie turned around to greet them.

"Guys, this is Halie. Halie, this is Kenny and Melinda."

"Hi. Jason's told me all about you," Halie responded.

"Well, Jason's a little quiet, so we look forward to spending some time getting to know you," Melinda replied. "Jane has kept us up to date."

"Yeah, Halie, it's like pulling teeth to get anything out of Jason," Kenny chimed in.

"Okay, let's stop the Jason-bashing," Jason said, as they pulled away.

"Jason, we can stay in a motel. You don't need to put us up," Melinda said.

"No way. You guys will be in the master bedroom. Besides, tomorrow, Halie's moving in, and we'll use you all as slave labor," Jason laughed.

"Jason, they don't need to help. I don't have that much."

"Hey, Jeff and I are taking the day off to move you, so I thought

Kenny and Melinda might like to hang out with us."

"Absolutely," Kenny responded.

Jason and Halie had already moved all of Halie's clothes and small articles into the guest quarters. All that remained to be moved was furniture. Most would be stored in the garage.

"Have you all been here before?" Jason asked, as they pulled up into the driveway.

"No. We were at your dad's house but never here," Melinda replied. "This looks like a castle."

"Yeah, I know. It's actually pretty spooky."

"It's a great old house," Halie commented. "Jason gave me a tour when we first met."

Jason parked behind the house and helped carry Kenny and Melinda's suitcases upstairs.

"Let's go out on the front porch and visit," he said, as he came down the stairs.

"Wow, the porch is bigger than our apartment," Melinda commented.

"Halie, Melinda, you all go out on the porch. I need to talk with Jason for a minute," Kenny remarked.

Kenny and Jason headed to the kitchen.

"What's up?" Jason asked.

"I found the housekeeper."

Chapter Sixty-Three

Jason could feel the hair on the back of his neck rise. He could feel the adrenaline pumping through his veins as he leaned forward. He hadn't expected Kenny to find the housekeeper. He had all but given up on the idea.

"Where is she?"

"She's in the same cemetery as Alyssa. Her name was Laynie Jessup."

"She's dead?" Jason asked.

"Yes, she died in 1957."

"Damn. How did you find her?"

"I made some assumptions based on what you told me. Using those assumptions, I did a computer search factoring in possible variables."

"I don't get it. What do you mean?"

"Okay, I tried to imagine what her life would've been like - where she would've lived, shopped, eaten, prayed, etc, etc. I found the roster of the Ebenezer Baptist Church that you told me about and researched the 23 names that appeared to be single females of the approximate age of the housekeeper. Eventually, I found her."

"Wow. What makes you so sure it's her?"

"Because I found the death certificate," Kenny replied.

"Why was that so important?"

"The certificate wasn't. The name of the doctor that signed it was. It was your grandfather."

"What did she die of?" Jason asked.

"A brain hemorrhage."

"I need to talk to Dan."

"Jason, you should also know that your grandfather paid for the cemetery plot. I checked the funeral-home records."

Jason sat quietly, trying to take in what Kenny was telling him. If Oliver had signed the death certificate, it meant he'd been with the housekeeper after his marriage to Miriam. It made no sense. One mystery had been solved, but others remained.

"Hey, can you stay here with Halie and Melinda while I run a quick errand?" Jason asked.

"Sure."

"I'll be back in an hour."

Jason called Dan and asked that he meet him in 15 minutes at Alyssa's grave. By the sound of his voice, Dan knew it was important. Driving to the cemetery, Jason felt exhilarated. For once, pieces were starting to fall together. When he arrived Dan was already standing at Alyssa's gravesite. The early-day fog had lifted, and sun shone through lingering clouds to give the cemetery a spring-like feel.

"What's the emergency? You pulled me away from a very hot encounter," Dan laughed.

"Come with me," Jason replied.

Dan was confused. He didn't know where Jason was headed. Walking four rows beyond Alyssa's grave, Jason stopped. He looked down on an average tombstone set under a tree.

"Who's this?" Dan asked.

"The housekeeper, Laynie Jessup."

"The housekeeper. The housekeeper we've been looking for?"

"One and the same. Kenny found her."

"How? We've been looking for the last month," Dan asked.

"You need to ask? Remember, it's Kenny. He can find anything."

"Wow, Laynie Jessup. She died young - 1957. Same year as the picture of her at the birthday party."

Jason looked at Dan.

"That's not the half of it. Guess who signed her death certificate?"

"Oliver?" Dan replied.

"Yes. Cause of death was listed as a brain hemorrhage."

"That means..."

"Yes, I know. He saw her after he was married to my grandmother. My dad was seven at the time."

Newly placed flowers set by the gravestone showed someone was caring for the grave.

"I wonder who put the flowers here? They look new. We know the cemetery doesn't put flowers out," Dan conjectured.

"Kenny told me Oliver also paid for the plot."

"Okay, if Oliver paid for the plot and signed the death certificate, he had to have seen her before she died, and he must have seen the little girl. He saw his daughter," Dan responded.

"Oh, shit. We've got to tell my dad. He's going to be floored."

"You know, I think this may be enough to get Menick to talk," Dan said, as he examined the flowers.

"Anything on the flowers?" Jason asked.

"No, except that they came from Cicero Florists. Wow, Cicero again. Seems like everything revolves around Cicero," Dan surmised.

"We need to tell my dad."

Dan looked back at the gravestone.

"Can we wait until the morning?"

"Sure. How about I meet you there at 8:00 a.m.? I'll call him tonight and tell him we need to talk."

"I'm going to stop at the florist on my way home. I'll let you know if I find anything," Dan promised.

Both men stopped at Alyssa's gravesite on the way out of the cemetery.

"You coming Sunday?" Jason asked.

"I'll be here. Jane's coming. We leave on the honeymoon at 4:00 p.m., so there should be plenty of time. How about you?"

"Halie and I will be here."

Driving to Cicero, Dan knew the answers to his questions resided with Frederick Menick. He drove 18 blocks out of the way in order to drive past both Bruno's and Frederick's homes.

"I'll see each of you again," he said aloud to himself.

The florist was still open. Dan arrived 30 minutes before closing.

"Are you the owner?" he said to the thin, elderly man.

"Yes, I'm Alfred Sandring. What can I do for you?"

Dan looked around the shop. It was small and old, and clearly had been the neighborhood florist for generations.

"I'm Dan Johnson, with the Chicago Police Department. I just have a couple questions I wanted to ask you."

"Sure - how can I help?"

"How long have you owned the shop?"

"Well, my father owned it before me. It's been in our family for 70 years. I've been running it for 30 years, ever since he died."

"Mr. Sandring, did you place flowers at the grave of Laynie Jessup in the Mt. Pleasant Cemetery? I found some with your label on them."

"Yes, I do every Monday morning. Why?" Alfred asked.

"How long have you been doing it?"

"My father started in 1957, and I still do today. When he died, he left very specific instructions. He told me a doctor set up an endowment to cover the costs of the flowers. His instructions were to place them for as long as our shop was open."

"But his name wasn't on the flowers," Dan continued.

"No, never is. Those were his instructions. My father gave him his word, and we live by our word."

As Dan drove back home, he called Jason.

"Jason, I just visited the florist."

"Find out anything?"

"Yes. Your grandfather set up an endowment at the florist in 1957. They've been placing the flowers on the grave every Monday morning."

"If he did that, and if he knew the child was his, it explains the $1,000-a-month deposit in Frederick's account. I think Oliver made those deposits to help support the child."

"That's a leap, but pretty reasonable."

"I think it's true," Jason replied.

"Why did they stop in 1999?" Dan asked.

"All I can guess is, it had to do with my grandmother's death. She died in 1999. I don't know what happened, but they stopped. By then, his daughter would have been 51 years old."

"Did Frederick still work for Oliver at that time?" Dan asked.

"Yes. There was so much more to my grandfather's relationship with Frederick than I or my dad ever knew. Frederick's the only one who can explain it all."

"Okay - see you tomorrow at 8:00 a.m. at your dad's, right?"

"Right."

Chapter Sixty-Four

By the time Jason got back to the house, Melinda, Kenny, and Halie had finished two bottles of wine. Jeff Dodson had joined them. Knowing that Melinda and Kenny were coming to town, he took a chance they'd all be gathered at Jason's. It was past 6:00 p.m. The time at the cemetery had slipped by.

"Hey, guys. Sorry I had to run out like that, but it was important."

"That's okay," Melinda replied. "We've been grilling Halie. She's held up real well."

Jason bent over and kissed Halie on the cheek.

"Hey, you can do better than that," Jeff kidded.

Jason turned back to Halie, pulled her out of her seat, and kissed her passionately.

"Now, have you sufficiently embarrassed my girlfriend?" Jason scolded.

Halie blushed.

"So, do you guys want to stay an extra day?" Jason asked, looking at Kenny and Melinda.

"We can't. We have to get back to class."

"What if I told you that on Monday you both have interviews for residencies at Cook County and Northwestern? You do well on the interview, you'll be here come July."

Kenny reached for his cell phone.

"What're you doing?" Jason asked.

"Calling the airline to reschedule."

"You'd better be. Heck, if we need to stay two days, it's fine by me," Melinda responded. "Thanks, Jason. How did you get that done?"

"Wasn't me. It was my dad. Thank him when you see him at the wedding."

For the next four hours, the friends shared their lives. Wine flowed, and, at 9:00 p.m., Jason called for three large pizzas.

"Hey, if anyone has had too much to drink tonight, you're staying with us. No arguments," Jason announced.

"Well, since I'm the only one who's not already staying here, I'll just accept your invitation right now," Jeff replied. "I'll take one of the bedrooms next to you and Halie. That way, you'll behave tonight."

Halie smiled and turned toward Jason. She'd only spent two nights in the house and still felt a little uncomfortable.

"Don't worry, Halie. You'll get used to Jeff's sense of humor."

Kenny motioned Jason into the house. He was curious about what he'd found at the cemetery.

"Was I right?"

"Yep. Laynie Jessup is buried there. She died in 1957, and, according to the people at the cemetery, Oliver bought her plot. It's all like you said. I can't believe I've been visiting that cemetery for more than four years and never knew."

Kenny handed him a beer.

"How could you have known? I just got lucky."

"No, Kenny, you're very good at what you do. We both know that. By the way - any luck on that safe-deposit box?"

"Not yet, but I'm working on it."

They rejoined the group on the porch as Melinda was pumping Jeff for information.

"So, Jeff. Tell me about Meredith. Jason's told us you kinda have a thing for her," Melinda queried.

Jeff looked at Jason with a frown.

"You weren't supposed to tell anyone about our visit."

"Hey, it's amongst friends," Jason replied.

"Come on, Jeff," Melinda prodded.

"Alright. I admit it I've had a crush on Meredith for a long time. I was just too chicken to act on it. Now, I think it's too late," he responded. Melinda wouldn't let it go. She was good at getting people to talk. Jason knew it when he told her about Jeff's crush.

"Why is it too late?" she asked.

"Because Meredith is with someone else now."

"Who is this guy?" she continued.

Jeff stood up and walked over to the steps. He didn't want to talk about it.

"Well," Melinda continued.

"Jason, you know. You tell her," Jeff replied.

Feeling his friend's uneasiness, Jason stepped forward.

"His name's Michael Grant. He'll be at the party tomorrow night."

"He's coming to the party?" Jeff asked.

"Yes, and don't you dare cancel," Jason replied.

"Oh, I'll be there. I'm looking forward to meeting him."

"Melinda, we don't know anything about this guy. Meredith met him in Aruba when she went there to celebrate graduation from residency. Every time we ask her about him, she shuts down. She's very protective of him."

"Maybe he's in the CIA," Kenny laughed.

"I doubt that, but just back off him for the party. Melinda, can you do that?" Jason stressed, looking at his friend.

"I'll try, but you know me. If he's really good looking, we may talk," Melinda laughed.

"Kenny, you okay with that?" Jeff asked.

"Heck, yes. I know at the end of the night she'll be chasing me around the bed. I have confidence in that," Kenny replied.

Laughter broke out. Kenny enjoyed watching other men admire his fiancée.

"You're right, sweetheart, so be ready," Melinda responded.

"Okay, now let's tone it down. Remember, guys, you all are in the guest quarters on the third floor. That's right above Halie and my bedroom, so keep it down."

"I thought we were going in the master bedroom," Melinda joked.

"You were - until I moved in. Sorry, guys," Halie responded.

"Halie, I was just kidding," Melinda replied.

"I know. Jason even replaced the old mattress in the master suite."

"I don't know how my grandfather slept on that thing," Jason laughed.

Jason had moved all of his clothing and belongings into the master suite on the second floor. Everything that had been in the closets had been moved to other bedrooms. Sometime in the future he would arrange for Goodwill to pick it all up. The first two nights with Halie in what had been his grandparent's room were eerie. Only Halie's presence next to him in bed allowed him to sleep. Her warmth gave him a secure feeling in what had been an uncomfortable place.

Halie enjoyed the banter taking place in front of her. Hearing Jason talk about the bedroom as theirs gave her a warm feeling. Kenny, Melinda, and Jeff were now her friends. She was part of their group.

"Hey, I hate to break this up, but we have a move to do tomorrow. We need to be sober when we pick up Halie's furniture," Jason commented.

"I second that," Halie chuckled.

Chapter Sixty-Five

With less than 24 hours remaining before his wedding, Dan was starting to feel nervous. He knew how great his life would be with Jane, but it was still an adjustment. As he pulled up in front of James's house, he decided to put his nerves aside. Jason had already arrived and was waiting on the sidewalk. James saw them approaching and came out on the front porch.

"Let's take a walk," he suggested.

Dan and Jason followed him.

"So what brings you here this morning? I know we'll all be back here tonight for the rehearsal, so it must be important," James asked.

"It is," Jason replied. "Dad, we found the housekeeper."

"Where is she? Is she still in Chicago?"

"No, she's dead. She died in 1957 from a brain hemorrhage," Jason replied.

"What was her name?"

"Laynie Jessup."

"What do we know?" James asked.

"We know grandfather signed her death certificate and that he bought her plot at the cemetery. We also know that, for the last 40 odd years, he's had a florist put flowers on her grave every Monday morning."

James stopped walking.

"That means he saw her after marrying your grandmother."

"Yes, but let's not jump to any conclusions about the relationship," Dan added.

"Well, we know he fathered her child," James responded.

Jason looked at Dan. Each was reluctant to go further.

"What are you not telling me? I can see it in your faces."

"Dad, she may have given birth to two babies. One, a boy, was stillborn, but it's possible - and I stress possible - that she gave birth to a little girl as well."

"You mean I might have a half-sister out there somewhere?" James asked.

"Maybe," Dan replied. "When I went back into Caseo's apartment the day we met with him, I found two pictures that were of interest. One was of him with a young woman and another taken at a birthday party on March 18, 1957. The group shot showed Bruno, Frederick, Frederick's mother, the housekeeper who we now know to have been Laynie Jessup, and a young girl. The nine candles on her cake indicate she was born the same day as the newspaper in the trunk was published."

"Then Bruno and Frederick know the truth. We need to talk to them."

"We talked to Frederick again. He shut down, but that was before Kenny found her name and what happened to her. Maybe now he'll open up," Jason replied.

"Where's she buried?" James asked.

"A stone's throw from Alyssa. All this time she was so close," Jason replied.

"You've talked to the florist and the cemetery to confirm this?"

"Yes, James. It's true," Dan reiterated.

"I want to see that picture. I also want to see the grave," James responded.

"Well, come to the cemetery with us Sunday, and we'll show you," Jason replied.

Victoria could see the three men talking on the sidewalk. She walked out on the front porch and called out.

"Dan, would you like to see the set-up for tomorrow?"

"Sure," Dan replied.

"Dad, Halie and I'll pick you up at 1:00 p.m. Sunday afternoon. Is that okay?" Jason asked.

"Yeah, sure. If I truly have a sister out there, I want to find her."

Victoria had spared no expense. The wedding would take place in the flower garden in back of the house. The reception would follow. The weather forecast for Chicago was for clear skies and temperatures in the mid-70s. The wedding was scheduled to start at 4:00 p.m. Caterers, florists, and those involved in the set-up would descend on the Conrad home at 7:00 a.m.

"What do you think? Will it work?" Victoria asked, knowing the answer.

"It's perfect. Tomorrow will be a great day," Dan replied.

"Now, remember, the rehearsal is at 5:00 p.m. today."

"I know. Trust me - we'll be here."

Jason chuckled as Dan followed Victoria around getting instructions.

"Don't laugh. I have a feeling you'll be doing this with Halie pretty soon," Dan whispered.

James sat in the den, sipping coffee. The idea that he had a sister had never entered his mind. Until now, it had been about the dead baby only. If she was his sister, she would be 62 years old now, he thought to himself. She could be anywhere. It was likely she either didn't exist, died, or lived elsewhere. Still, he wanted to know.

His search for the safe-deposit box now extended 30 miles from Hinsdale. As of yet, he had no results. He was getting discouraged. The morning paper sat next to him on the desk. The headlines on the front page took him to another place and time. "Alphonse and Anthony Savuzzo Indicted" read the lead headline of the *Chicago Tribune*. James sat up in his chair and continued to read. A picture of Lisbeth Williams, Jane's new boss, was inserted below the copy. According to the article, both Al and Tony had been arrested for extortion, money laundering, assault, battery, and arson. The charges all stemmed from accusations made by three merchants in downtown Chicago who claimed they were threatened and physically assaulted by Savuzzo thugs. An unnamed source had provided information that led to the arrests. Williams was in charge of the case.

"Can I talk to Dan for a minute?" James asked as he interrupted

Victoria's tour.

"Sure, I'll get Jason some coffee."

"You mind, Jason?" James asked.

"No, go ahead."

Dan followed James out to the front porch.

"You see this?" James asked, showing Dan the newspaper.

"No, but Jane told me last night it was coming."

"Do you think this unnamed source is Bruno Caseo?"

"Yes, I do. Remember? He said he had someone he knew in the DA's office. I think he may already have talked to them when we came by."

"Do you think this will lead to me?"

Dan looked at the floor.

"I don't know James. I wish I knew."

"Did Jane say whether it was a solid case?"

"She said Williams doesn't get indictments unless she's sure she can get a conviction."

Jason walked out on the front porch just as Dan and James were finishing. He could tell that his father was disturbed about something. As soon as James left, he turned to Dan.

"I didn't realize this would hit him this hard."

Dan pulled out the newspaper.

"It wasn't just the news about Laynie Jessup and her daughter," Dan said, as he opened the paper to the story about the Savuzzos.

"Damn, this couldn't have happened at a worse time," Jason commented.

"Yeah, I know."

"I bet my dad's worried this could lead to Oliver."

"All we can do is hope it doesn't," Dan replied, knowing that James' main concern was that it might lead to Leonard Simpson - and to him.

Chapter Sixty-Six

The luster of the weekend had been muted. Dan could feel the stress and tension in James. He knew it would eventually impact Jason. Jason had become like a son to him. He wanted to protect him. He smiled as he saw Jane sitting at the kitchen table.

"Hey, sweetheart," Jane said, kissing him as he entered the kitchen. A *Chicago Tribune* lay open on the table.

"I see you've already read the paper. What did you think about the indictments?"

"All I know is she must have some good information," Jane responded.

"Yeah, and I think I know where it's coming from."

"Really? Who?"

"Can I talk to you as my fiancée, not as a cop or a DA?"

"Sure, you know what you tell me is private unless you say otherwise."

"Jason and I have been working on something off the record. It involves his family. One of the keys to the case is a long-time Savuzzo bodyguard. He has a wealth of information, some of it written down. He said he had a contact in the DA's office. I think he's the source of what's happening."

"What are you working on?" Jane pressed.

Dan hesitated. He didn't want to start the marriage with deception. He felt like he could trust Jane's discretion.

"In this room, right?"

"Yes, you know that."

"Jason found the remains of a stillborn child in a trunk in his grandfather's house. He and James have been trying to find out who the baby was and how it got there. They brought me into it about a month ago. I haven't reported it yet."

"Dan, you know the risk you're taking?"

"I know, but I had to give them some time to unravel it."

"You've got to report it. You could lose your job over this," Jane responded.

"I will, soon."

"How close are you to solving it?"

"Very close, I think. We've found the mother. Unfortunately, she's dead. We have several very good leads that I think will pan out in the next couple weeks."

"Do you want to postpone the honeymoon?"

"No way. Jason can handle it without me for a few days. He'll call me if he needs me," Dan replied. "Let's change the subject. This is supposed to be a happy time. Tomorrow, we get married."

He pulled her into his arms and held her tightly. He could feel her warm body underneath her robe. She looked up into his eyes and kissed him.

"I think we need to spend a bit more time in the bedroom this morning. That okay with you?" Jane whispered.

When Jason returned, Halie had already fixed Kenny and Melinda breakfast. They were sitting around the dining room table, talking about medical school. Halie and Melinda were in robes, Kenny in shorts and a tee shirt. Jason looked at Halie and smiled.

"Hey, what are you smiling at?" Halie said as Jason sat down.

"I don't know. I guess this just really feels good. It feels like you're supposed to be here."

Halie got up and went over to him and wrapped her arms around his neck. She kissed his forehead and pulled a chair up next to him.

"Where's Jeff? Let me guess. He's still asleep."

"Actually no. He left 30 minutes ago to go get a truck for the move. He's been up for a couple hours. I think he's having a hard time sleeping, thinking about seeing Meredith tonight," Halie replied.

"Where are Meredith and this new guy staying?" Kenny asked.

"With Claire and Jackson, I think. Maybe they'll be able to give us a read on him after they leave. Melinda, you're quiet this morning," Jason observed.

"I'm always quiet in the morning. You've seen me plenty of times in the morning. You've forgotten med school," Melinda responded.

"Actually I've tried to forget."

"My time's the night. I thrive at night," Melinda replied.

"Yeah, and mine's the morning. We're a great match, aren't we?" Kenny laughed. "We're the opposite in everything. I think that's why we get along so well."

Thirty minutes later, Jeff drove up the driveway with a rental truck. Quickly, Jason and Kenny changed. The drive to Halie's took 20 minutes. It was a perfect day to move. The weather had cooperated for both the move and the wedding. Halie and Jason had already packed all the boxes, so moving involved only loading and unloading the truck. Halie and Melinda stayed behind. As the truck pulled out, they took cups of coffee out to the front porch. It would be their time. Melinda had wanted to spend some private time with Jason's new love.

"Halie, I haven't seen Jason this happy in a long time."

"I haven't been, either. Maybe the time was right," Halie replied.

"Dan told us you've been to the cemetery."

"Yes, I go with Jason every couple of weeks. Sometimes I stay home. I think sometimes he needs that time on his own."

"Wow - you're amazing. That takes a great deal of depth," Melinda said shaking her head.

Over the next hour, Melinda told Halie how she and Kenny had gotten involved in Jason's life. She left nothing out. She spoke about Alyssa, medical school, the investigation, the aftermath, and where they were today. It gave Halie a sense of comfort knowing Jason had such loyal friends.

"Jason's lucky to have you and Kenny."

"Hey, he's lucky to have you," Melinda replied.

"I'm worried about his friend Jeff. I wish there was something I could do."

"We can help. At least we can check out who this Michael Grant is. We owe Jeff and Jason that. Kenny can do a background search, and I have my ways of finding out how legit someone is," Melinda laughed.

"Hey, Jason told me about what you did with that Physiology professor at your medical school. Don't be taking any risks like that again, okay?"

"I won't. I'll be careful. I know the limits I can push," Melinda responded.

Melinda had already decided she was going to test Michael Grant at the party. She knew she could tell how earnest he was about Meredith.

"Good luck on your interviews Monday. It sure would be great to have you in Chicago. We don't have many friends to socialize with."

"Thanks. Jason's dad really came through for us. It's another reason to make sure Meredith doesn't get hurt."

It took only an hour and a half to load the truck. When they returned, Jason backed it up into the driveway.

"Okay, we got it here. Now you ladies have to unload it,' Jeff called out.

"Funny man," Melinda yelled back. "In your dreams."

Melinda gave back as well as she took banter. Jeff knew he'd met his match.

"Where do you want all of this?" Jeff asked.

"I'll show you," Jason replied as he, Jeff, and Kenny walked back to the garage.

He'd cleared half of the garage for the furniture. He and Halie would decide later what to do with it.

"What's under the tarp?" Jeff asked.

"You never saw my grandfather's car?"

"No, take the tarp off," Jeff replied.

Jason untied the ends of the tarp and pulled it off the car.

"Oh my god," Kenny exclaimed. "A 1939 Caddy convertible with leather interior and electric windows. This is a classic."

"I didn't know you knew so much about cars," Jason commented.

"My hobby. I just never had time for it in med school. In high school and college, I spent a lot of time tinkering. I wasn't exactly Mr. Big on campus, so I had a lot of time to myself."

"Kenny, you're a great friend. If not for you, we would never have tracked down Alyssa's killers," Jason said, as he reached for the car keys hanging on a peg-board next to the car.

With a quick motion he tossed the keys to Kenny.

"As of today, it's yours."

"What are you talking about? This car's worth more than $100,000. You can't just give it away," Kenny replied.

"Is it mine?" Jason asked.

"Yes."

"Then I can give it away. I just did. It's now your car. Check it out. Drive it back to North Carolina."

"You heard the man. It's your car now, so stop hogging space in Jason's garage," Jeff laughed.

Kenny was shocked. He didn't believe what he was hearing.

"Jason, I can't accept this. It's not right."

"Kenny, you, Melinda, and Jeff are my best friends. You were Alyssa's friends. I want to do this because I know she would have wanted me to. Don't ruin the moment by refusing. Please accept it with my gratitude."

"Mind if I get Melinda?" Kenny asked.

"No, go ahead," Jason replied.

Kenny went inside. Jeff nodded at Jason.

"You're one hell of a guy, my friend."

"Jeff, so are you. True friends are those you can count on, no matter what. I count you, Kenny, and Melinda as mine."

"Okay, so where's my car?" Jeff laughed. "Just kidding. I don't like old cars anyway. I'm more into a new Lexus or Mercedes; so, if you come across one of those, let me know."

Melinda came out to the garage with Kenny.

"Thanks Jason, but we can't accept it," Melinda said, as she walked around the car.

"Why?"

"Because it's dirty. You're going to wash it first, right?"

"Of course. I wouldn't want you guys driving a dirty car back home. The people in Wilmington might not let you in."

"Okay, I hate to break this up, but we need to get going. The rehearsal's in four hours. You also have a party to get ready for," Jeff commented.

It only took an hour to unload. Once finished, everyone moved inside to get ready to go to James and Victoria's for the rehearsal. Halie would be staying behind to get ready for the party. Guests would be arriving between 6:00 p.m. and 7:00 p.m. By 4:30 p.m., everyone had left for the rehearsal. Halie was alone, preparing for the party. At 6:00 p.m. she heard a knock at the door. Rounding the corner, she saw a tall, older man standing on the porch.

"May I help you?"

"Is Jason Conrad in, by chance?"

"No, but he'll be back soon."

"My name's Frederick Menick. Will you tell him I came by and that I'd like to talk to him?"

"Sure. I'll have him call you."

"Thank you very much," Frederick replied, as he turned to walk away.

He stopped at the end of the sidewalk and looked at the house he'd spent a lifetime in. Memories flooded back. He could see Oliver, Miriam,

James, and Laynie. His best and worst memories had been in Oliver Conrad's home. He started to cry as he turned away once more.

Chapter Sixty-Seven

The rehearsal at the Conrad home went smoothly. The atmosphere was light and full of happiness. Only James, who stayed inside most of the time, showed any sign that his mind was elsewhere. It had been a difficult three years for Dan. Jason was intent on making sure that the wedding and everything around it was positive. The same pastor who had married Jason and Alyssa would be conducting the ceremony. Even during rehearsal, Victoria cried.

"Alright, that's over. Now, let's go party," Jason commented as he said goodbye to his mother and father.

Kenny and Melinda had ridden with Jason. They all piled into Jason's car. Dan and Jane followed them back to Jason's house. When they got there, several vehicles were parked out front. Jason could make out Jeff's and Claire's. Halie greeted him at the front door.

"You had a visitor while you were gone," Halie told Jason as he walked in.

"Really? Who?"

"A man named Frederick Menick. He said he needed to talk to you."

Frederick Menick, Jason thought to himself. *What would he want?*

"He gave me his phone number and asked that you call."

"Thanks, babe. I'll call him right now."

Jason waited for Dan and Jane to arrive.

"Jane, may I borrow him for a second?" Jason asked.

"Sure - just bring him back."

They headed to the corner of the porch.

"What's up?" Dan asked.

"Frederick Menick came by while I was gone. He wants me to call him."

"He must want to talk," Dan replied.

Pulling out his cell phone, Jason dialed Frederick's number.

"Hello," Frederick answered.

"Frederick, this is Jason Conrad. I had a message to call you."

"Jason, can you come by and visit me tomorrow?"

"Sure. I have a wedding to attend, but I could stop by tomorrow morning – say, around 9:00 a.m. Would that work?"

"That would be fine. I'll see you tomorrow," Frederick closed.

"You want to go?" Jason asked Dan.

"Yeah. I'm not supposed to see Jane tomorrow anyway until the wedding. I'll be staying at the Marriott on Michigan Avenue tonight. Can you pick me up at 8:30 a.m.?"

"Sure," Jason replied.

Jane had waited with Halie in the foyer.

"Who's here?" Jason asked as he came back inside.

"Claire and Jackson are here. So are Jeff, Bill, and Melissa," Halie replied.

"How about Meredith?"

"They just got here. I think they're in the kitchen."

"Okay, I'll make my rounds and say hi," he replied.

Dan and Jane walked into the parlor. Bill, Jason's older brother, knew Dan from Alyssa's wedding and funeral, but hadn't met Jane.

"Jane, this is Bill and Melissa. Bill is Jason's big brother. He's a cardiologist in Chicago. I guess I should say he's my cardiologist."

"Hi, Jane. It's a pleasure to meet you," Bill replied.

"Does Dan have a heart problem?"

"No, actually it was an ulcer, but it was wise to check it out. Alyssa insisted."

"Melissa, I hear you have three children. Victoria must be very pleased."

"Yes, she is. Now we have another future Conrad on the way, with Claire's pregnancy," Melissa responded.

Jane felt at home. The Conrad family was welcoming and hospitable. Jason and Halie walked over to Claire and Jackson.

"Hi, Claire. Have you met Halie?"

"No, and I'm pissed that you haven't introduced us. You cancelled the dinner plans we had several weeks ago. I'm holding you to that rain check you asked for."

"We'll go, trust me," Jason replied. "Claire, did you find out anything when you canvassed the neighborhood? I meant to ask you last week."

"No, everybody's died who would've known anything."

Halie listened. She didn't understand what they were referring to. Jason knew he needed to tell her what was going on.

"Jason, have you taken Halie to brunch with Mom and Dad yet?" Claire asked.

"No Claire, but we will, soon."

Jason leaned close to Halie and whispered.

"I'm sorry. I meant to take you to dinner with my folks and with Claire, but it's just been so busy."

"That's alright. I'd love to meet them."

"You will, sweetheart. I promise."

Jason could see Meredith in the dining room. Dressed in a short skirt and open blouse, she had taken off her glasses and was wearing spiked heels. It wasn't the Meredith that he knew.

"That must be Michael," he whispered to Halie.

"Your sister's a knockout. You didn't tell me she was so pretty. The guy's not bad looking, either," Halie replied.

"Hey, watch it. You're taken," Jason chuckled.

Meredith had told them that Michael Grant was in his late 30s. He had short blond hair and was of medium height. He was a good-looking man, someone who wouldn't have trouble attracting women. The look on Meredith's face as she talked to him told Jason how infatuated she was. She hung on his every word. As he spoke, her eyes focused on him and no one else.

"Okay, here goes. I'm going to introduce myself. Wanna come?"

"No. I already met them, but you go ahead," Halie replied.

Before he could get to Meredith, Melinda stepped in between. Kenny was in the den, talking to Bill about the cardiology program he would be interviewing for. Melinda had gone upstairs to change after returning from the rehearsal. She knew Michael Grant would be at the party. She intended to test him. The look on his face when she talked to him or to others would tell her a great deal. Where his eyes focused and the body language he exhibited would tell her if he was genuine about his feelings for Meredith. Even Jason was stunned by what Melinda wore. The sheer white linen blouse showed ample cleavage. The slit mini skirt and pump heels made him look twice. Melinda's long blond hair fell over her shoulders, highlighting her blue eyes. Jason quickly turned around and headed back to Halie.

"Do you see what Melinda has on?"

"Oh yeah. I noticed. I think everyone noticed. My guess is she wants to see if Michael notices," Halie responded.

"I'm gonna go see Kenny."

Jason found Kenny in the den. Interrupting his conversation with Bill, he pulled him into the parlor.

"Kenny, have you seen Melinda?"

"Yeah, why?"

"You're alright with what she's wearing?" Jason asked.

"Sure, she looks hot, doesn't she? And to think she'll be going home with me tonight - or should I say upstairs - with me tonight," Kenny laughed.

"What's she doing?" Jason asked.

"Testing Michael. She says she can tell by his reaction whether he's sincere."

"Great. Unfortunately, you'd have to be a monk not to look at her. She's pretty well all out there. I think every guy in here tonight's gonna get in trouble."

Melinda wasted no time.

"Hi, I'm Melinda," she said, shaking Michael's hand.

"Nice to meet you," Michael replied.

She maintained the handshake, wanting him to feel the touch of her skin. She could sense Meredith's uneasiness.

"Hi, Meredith. We met a few years ago," Melinda said, turning to her.

"Yes, I remember you, Melinda. You went to school with Jason, right?"

"Yes, I'm finishing this year. Your dad set up an interview for me Monday with Cook County. I'm going into Orthopedic Surgery," Melinda answered.

"Aren't you dating someone here?" Meredith asked.

"Yes, Kenny; he's in the den. He's going into Cardiology."

Melinda moved closer to Michael. Without anyone noticing, she pressed against his arm. She knew he could feel her breasts. He didn't move away. He stayed in contact with her. Turning toward Meredith, she made sure to watch him out of the corner of her eye. When Meredith looked away, he scanned up and down Melinda's body as if to examine a potential purchase.

"Hey, it was great meeting you," Melinda said, as she walked away toward the bar in the kitchen.

Kenny stood in the hallway, watching. Melinda had given him specific instructions as to what to look for. It didn't take long to spot what she knew would happen. Michael, when the opportunity existed and Meredith wasn't watching, turned to watch Melinda walk away. As soon as he did, Kenny walked over to Meredith and asked if he could talk to her. She obliged and followed him into the den. Moments later, Michael headed to the kitchen to see Melinda.

"So, you're a friend of Jason's. He owns this house, right?" Michael asked.

"Yes, we've been friends for about four years. Are you dating his sister?" Melinda asked.

"Yes, we met in Aruba and have been seeing each other. She's a really sweet gal."

For the next 10 minutes Michael and Melinda engaged in small talk. Melinda made sure to touch him on his arm or his hand throughout the discussion. She watched as he examined her body at every opportunity. Twice, she caught him staring at her breasts.

"There you are, baby," Kenny said, as he came into the kitchen.

"Hi, Kenny; this is Michael. We were just getting to know each other," she answered.

"Good to meet you, Michael. Sorry I took Meredith away. She's looking for you."

Jeff had watched the entire interlude. He didn't say anything, but he felt certain that Michael was trying to make inroads with Melinda.

"Meredith, got a minute?" Jeff asked as Meredith searched for Michael.

"Sure, Jeff. How you been?"

"Good. Things are going pretty well. Looks like you're doing well. You look beautiful."

"Thanks, Jeff. Yes, I'll be moving back to Chicago soon. I'm so glad to be done with residency. Now, maybe I can earn a living."

"Well, your parents have to be very proud of you," Jeff told her.

"So, who are you here with?" Meredith asked.

"Nobody. Just me. I see you're dating someone. You like him?"

"Yes, I do. He's been really good for me. I just need to find him."

"I think I saw him go in the kitchen with Melinda," Jeff replied.

"Okay. It was good to see you," Meredith responded, as she walked away quickly toward the kitchen.

"I don't have a chance," Jeff said aloud to himself.

Chapter Sixty-Eight

The party went on past midnight. Bill and Melissa were the first to leave. With three small children, staying out late wasn't practical. Claire, now four months pregnant, left with Jackson soon thereafter. Jane and Dan called it a night at 11:00 p.m. Jane dropped Dan off at the Marriott and headed to her new home. Meredith and Michael left near midnight. They had a room at the Four Seasons Hotel downtown. Michael had insisted. He preferred not to stay at the cheaper Marriott or with Claire and Jackson.

Kenny and Melinda joined Jeff, Jason, and Halie on the front porch. Melinda excused herself to put something warmer on.

"I wondered if you were a bit chilly," Jason laughed.

"Ha ha, funny man. I had a reason to dress like I did. Besides, Kenny was impressed. That's all that matters," Melinda replied.

"Hey, you weren't supposed to be looking," Halie kidded, looking at Jason.

"How could you not look? Any guy would look."

"Michael did a lot more than look," Melinda said, as she returned in a sweat suit.

"Wow - that's a change. I think you went from covering very little to covering everything," Jeff commented.

"Listen, I know guys, and, if Meredith hadn't been here, that guy would have been all over me."

"He'd have to have gotten past me first," Kenny responded.

Melinda moved to Kenny's chair and sat on his lap. She wrapped her arms around him and kissed him.

"You know you're the only man for me," Melinda whispered.

"So, what do we do?" Jeff asked.

"Nothing, Jeff. She has to see it for herself," Jason replied.

At 2:30 a.m. they called it a night. Jason and Halie headed to their room.

"Who was that man who came by earlier?" Halie asked.

Jason decided it was time to tell her what was going on. He spent the next hour explaining what he found and what was being done. When he finished, Halie knew how important Frederick was to the case. Holding her close to him in bed, Jason found it difficult to sleep. His thoughts were on his meeting in a few hours and what it would divulge.

As predicted, it was a beautiful Saturday morning in Chicago. *Traffic will be light going downtown,* Jason thought to himself. The remnants of the party could still be seen on the porch. Driving through the neighborhood, he tried to imagine a time 60 years ago, when his grandparents would have been walking down the sidewalk, and his father would have been playing in the yard. As he passed what had been the home of Stillwell Jordan, he saw a new family moving in. Three small children were scurrying about the yard, investigating their new home. The thought of what his children with Alyssa might have looked like entered his mind. The honk of the horn behind him at the stop sign brought him back.

Dan was waiting on the curb outside the Marriott when Jason pulled up.

"Ready for the big day?"

"Ready as I'll ever be," Dan replied.

"I guess my job is to get you to the wedding on time. By the way, you haven't given me the ring yet. Aren't I supposed to hold it for you?"

Dan reached into his pocket and pulled out the ring.

"Watch over it. You lose it, you buy another," Dan laughed.

"Don't worry. I won't lose it."

"So, how did the rest of the party go?"

"Pretty well. We stayed up until 2:30 a.m., talking."

"So what was with Melinda? She sure got attention," Dan asked.

"Yeah, well it was her way of testing the sincerity of Michael Grant. You know Melinda. She has her own ways of finding things out."

"I know. I remember that Physiology prof at UA. He never had a chance. Once Melinda sets her mind to something, she makes it happen," Dan observed. "Was Kenny okay with it?"

"He loved it. He's very proud and very secure. She's totally in love with him."

"What was her conclusion?"

"She's pretty sure he's not legit. I guess he followed her into the kitchen, and enough happened that she and Kenny are convinced he's a player."

The drive to Frederick's house took 20 minutes. As they pulled up in front, Frederick was sitting on his front porch.

"Hope you don't mind, but I brought Dan with me. I know you've met before," Jason called out as they walked up the sidewalk.

"Do I have a choice? Sorry, Mr. Johnson, but I had expected only Jason."

"I can wait in the car," Dan replied.

"No, come in. You may as well hear this."

The three men walked into the house and took seats in the living room.

"I hear you're getting married today," Frederick said to Dan.

"Yes, in about six hours."

"Congratulations."

"Thank you."

As they talked, Jason scanned the room. The picture that had been removed was back in its place.

"What would you like to talk about, Frederick?" Jason asked.

"I know you went to the cemetery and that you found Laynie. The people at the cemetery called me."

"Yes, we found her gravesite. It's close to Alyssa's. We also know that my grandfather signed the death certificate and that he paid for the cemetery plot. He also set up a fund at Cicero Florist to place flowers on her grave every Monday morning. My guess is that the $1,000-a-month deposit in your account was made by him as well."

Frederick looked outside. He felt relief that finally someone else knew.

"Yes, Oliver signed the death certificate and bought the plot," Frederick replied.

He looked at the picture on the mantel and thought of the day when Oliver came to check on Laynie. It had been 54 years, but he remembered it like it was yesterday.

Chapter Sixty-Nine

May 1957

"Come in, Oliver," Frederick said as he opened the door.

Oliver reached out and grabbed the door molding. He felt unstable. Slowly, he entered the Menick home. Sophie stood in the middle of the room.

"Sophie, this is Dr. Conrad. He's come to see your mom."

Sophie extended her hand. She was shy around adults she didn't know.

"Glad to meet you, Dr. Conrad."

Oliver shook her hand thinking how strange it was to be introduced to his own child.

"Where's Laynie?" he asked.

"Follow me," Frederick replied.

Walking down the hallway, Oliver felt his hands shaking.

"Laynie, we have a visitor," Frederick said, as he opened the door.

The room was dark. Light bothered her eyes. Even so, there was enough light coming in through the doorway and a slit in the window for Oliver to see her and for her to see him.

"Oliver, you didn't have to come."

"Yes, I did. I don't know what to say. I'm so sorry."

"That's the past. Let's let that go and concentrate on the present," Laynie replied.

"Is Sophie my daughter?"

"Yes, she is."

"She's beautiful. She looks just like her mother."

"Thank you. She's also very smart, like her father. Top of her class."

"You've done a good job with her. I'm sorry I let you both down," he responded, trying to hold back tears.

"Oliver, please - let's not go back. It can't be changed. I'm happy that you found someone and that you have a beautiful son."

Oliver nodded his head.

"Frederick tells me you've been feeling bad. What seems to be the problem?"

Laynie told him about what she was experiencing. As she described her symptoms, Oliver felt a deep concern.

"We need to get you to a hospital and run some tests."

"No hospitals! Please."

"Laynie, without the tests, I won't know what's wrong," Oliver explained.

"We'll do it tomorrow if we must. Right now, I'm tired, and I just want to go to sleep."

"Tomorrow, then. I'll be here at 8:00 a.m. sharp," Oliver replied.

As he rose to leave, Laynie extended her hand to touch him. He reached down and grabbed her hand.

"Oliver, I'm sorry I left. It wasn't because I didn't love you. I just knew it wouldn't work. I didn't want to see you hurt."

"I know, Laynie. I just wish things had been different. I wish I'd had been better."

He leaned forward and kissed her on the forehead. Sophie was waiting in the living room.

"Frederick, can I talk to you for a minute on the porch?"

"Sure."

The two men walked outside. Gertrude, who had been doing dishes in the kitchen, came out and sat with Sophie.

"I think this is really serious. We need to get her into the hospital as soon as possible. I'm going to have an ambulance here tomorrow at 8:00 a.m. Have Gertrude take Sophie to the park, so she doesn't see it."

"Okay. What do you think it is?"

"I won't know until we see her tests."

Oliver shook hands with Frederick and left. He decided to avoid seeing Sophie again. He knew, if he did, it would be even harder to leave.

Miriam had gone to bed by the time he returned. As he walked down the hallway toward their room, he stepped inside James's room and approached the bed. He knelt down and kissed his son on the cheek.

"Everything okay?" Miriam asked, as he lay down next to her.

"I just had to go see a patient. They aren't doing too well. I'm sorry I was late."

"That's okay. James was tired, so we both went to bed early."

"I love you, Miriam," Oliver said, as he kissed her gently.

At 4:30 a.m., the house phone rang. Oliver got up and went downstairs to answer.

"Hello, hello, this is Dr. Conrad."

"Oliver, she's gone," Frederick replied.

Oliver knew what he meant. It was too late.

"Oliver, are you there?"

"Yes, Frederick, I'm here," he responded after several moments of silence.

"I got up to check on her 30 minutes ago and I couldn't wake her. She died in her sleep."

"Have you called anyone?" Oliver asked.

"No, just you."

"I'll be right over."

Sitting down on a chair next to the phone, Oliver began to cry. He couldn't believe Laynie was gone. He'd seen her for the first time in more than nine years just eight hours before. Now she was gone. Miriam could hear him talking on the phone.

"Is everything okay?" she called out from the landing.

Oliver composed himself and came to the foot of the steps.

"No, a patient of mine just died. I need to go arrange for the transfer and sign the death certificate. I'll be gone for a few hours."

"I'm so sorry. Anything I can do?"

"No; just take care of James. I'll be back soon."

The drive to Frederick's gave Oliver time to reflect on the past. He thought about the good times and the passion. Laynie had been part of his life for more than 30 years. She knew him better than anyone else. He blamed himself for the weakness that prevented him from recognizing their love publicly. His words hurt her. He tried to imagine what it had to feel like hearing him deny her to Stillwell Jordan. He knew the guilt of what he did would be with him until his dying breath. At the same time, he loved Miriam and James. He never wanted to hurt them. He would protect them at all cost.

As he approached Frederick's house, he thought of Sophie. The loss of her mother would devastate her. Thankfully, Frederick and Gertrude would be there to care for her. He wished he had the strength to recognize her as his and give her a home. He knew it would destroy his family. The only thing he could do was to ensure she was cared for and that her financial needs were met.

Chapter Seventy

Present Day

"Frederick, are you okay?" Jason asked, breaking Frederick's stare.

"I'm sorry. I was just thinking about the night Laynie died."

"What happened?" Dan asked.

"Laynie had left Oliver years before. I told him about where she was only because she was sick. He came over the night before she died. He arranged for an ambulance to pick her up and take her to the hospital the next morning for some tests. He wanted her to go that night, but she refused. She never made it to the next day. I found her and called Oliver. He came right over and called an ambulance. They took her to Cook County, where he signed the death certificate. She died of a brain hemorrhage."

"And everything after that?" Jason asked.

"Oliver took care of it all. We all swore ourselves to secrecy. Oh, and you're wrong about the $1,000-a-month deposit."

"How so?" Jason asked.

"Oliver made sure Sophie was cared for and that all her needs were met, but he didn't send the extra money."

"Who did?"

"Your grandmother. Oliver never knew. She sent the money with specific instructions about how to invest it."

"I don't understand. How did Miriam know?" Dan asked.

"She followed me one Sunday to my house. I think she was just curious about where I lived. She sat out front and saw Laynie and Sophie. When I got back, she confronted me, and I told her the story."

"What did she say?" Jason pressed.

"Nothing. It was as if she understood everything. She never spoke of it again. The first time she sent the money, she sent a note with it that it was to be placed in an account for Sophie."

Dan looked at Jason.

"What happened to the money?"

"Twelve years ago, when Miriam died, I told Sophie about the account. It had more than three million dollars in it. She instructed me to give it to Cook County Hospital to endow a chair in Neurology. She wanted to help others who might have the same affliction as her mother. If you go into the Neurology Department, you'll find a plaque hung in her mother's memory."

"So, Sophie's alive today. Does she know Oliver was her father?"

"No, she never will. That was Oliver's wish. If you hadn't pursued this I wouldn't be telling you this now."

Dan hesitated.

"What about the baby in the trunk?"

Frederick felt the blood drain from his face. He started to breathe heavy. Sweat started to roll off his forehead, and his left arm started to ache.

"Trunk," he said, as he collapsed on to the floor.

"Call 911, Dan. I think he's having a heart attack."

Dan quickly called for help. Within minutes, the EMT squad had arrived. While they waited, Jason administered CPR to the stricken Menick. Frederick reached up and grabbed Jason's hand.

"You don't understand, you don't understand," were his last words before he drifted into unconsciousness.

Dan and Jason backed away to let the EMTs work. After 15 minutes of CPR and several attempts to revive him with electric shock, they loaded him into the ambulance to take him to the hospital. The lead EMT turned to Jason and shook his head.

"I don't think he's going to make it."

"Oh, my God. I think that last question gave him a heart attack," Jason said, sitting down in a chair on the Menick porch.

"You don't know that, Jason," Dan replied.

The sounds of the ambulance brought Bruno Caseo out of his apartment. In minutes, he and four armed men were standing on Frederick's porch.

"What happened? Is Frederick okay? I could hear the ambulances," he asked.

Dan and Jason noticed the men around him. Dan recognized Joe Hansen. Hansen had been in his squad at Precinct 71, 15 years before. Now he was assigned to the DA's office.

"He had a heart attack. It's bad. They took him to Cook County," Dan replied.

"I need to go there," Bruno said, turning to Hansen.

"We can't. It's too unprotected," Hansen responded.

"Hey, Joe, how you been?" Dan asked.

"Fine - you?"

"Great; getting married today."

"Congratulations," Hansen answered, as he escorted Bruno to the car.

As quickly as they got there, Bruno and his bodyguards were gone. Jason motioned Dan to come inside the house.

"I guess we know now where the information came from to indict Al and Tony," Dan surmised.

"Yeah, Bruno must have been talking to his contact in the DA's office."

"Do you think Bruno's at risk?" Jason asked.

"Absolutely. Al will put out a hit on him if he hasn't already done so. Remember the indictments are of both Al and Tony."

"Look at this picture. Is that the same person you saw in the picture at Bruno's?"

"That's her - Laynie Jessup."

"Do you think Menick put the baby in the trunk?" Jason asked.

Walking around the room, looking at old pictures, Dan considered it.

"I think he did. I think Laynie gave birth to twins, and one died. Frederick probably panicked and did what he did. I wonder if Laynie ever knew she had given birth to twins."

"When I was in med school, I read an article once about midwifery. Apparently midwives in the black neighborhoods used a drug called Pethidine. It was used to disorient the patient so they could deal with the pain. Maybe the midwife knew one of the babies was dead and didn't want Laynie to know."

Dan paused to consider Jason's suggestion.

"Makes sense. That would explain Frederick's actions. He had to act quickly. He had to make sure Laynie never knew."

"We need to find Sophie Jessup," Jason replied.

"And we need to go over and tell your father about what just happened," Dan responded.

Chapter Seventy-One

Jason called the hospital on their way to see James. The hospital confirmed that Frederick had been admitted and was in critical condition in the intensive care unit. As they parked, they could see dozens of workers getting things ready for the wedding.

"Hard to get in the wedding mood after that," Dan commented.

"You will. There's nothing we can do about the past. Just enjoy the day. Once we tell James, we'll put this aside and concentrate on giving Jane a wonderful wedding," Jason responded.

"That would be nice."

James was sitting on the porch, reading the paper. It was a beautiful day to be outside. He was enjoying the sunshine.

"What brings the groom and best man over so early? Wedding doesn't start for a good while," James remarked.

"Dad, we just got back from seeing Frederick Menick. He came by the house yesterday and asked me to stop by and talk to him. Dan went with me."

"He tell you anything new?" James asked.

"Yes, he did, but before we were able to finish, and just after we asked about the baby in the trunk, he had a massive heart attack. He's in critical condition at Cook County. We just got the confirmation from the hospital."

"Frederick?"

"Yes."

"Damn - he was a good man. I felt sorry for him because he always seemed so alone," James replied.

Jason proceeded to tell his father about their visit. He explained how Frederick had confirmed the housekeeper's identity and how she died.

"So, Oliver did have a child with her?"

"Twins - we think one lived and one died. The one who lived, the little girl, moved with Laynie into Frederick's home. Frederick and his mother took care of them. Bruno Caseo fell in love with Frederick's sister, but she died early in 1958, soon after Laynie."

"How do we know her daughter - my sister - is alive?"

"Well, we know that, in 1999, she gave Cook County Hospital three million dollars to endow a Neurology Chair."

"Wait a minute. You mean the Jessup Chair of Neurology? I've known about that endowment for years. That was Oliver's housekeeper?"

"Yes. What you don't know is that the funds came from Grandmother. She had been sending Frederick $1,000 each month to put in a fund for Sophie. When she died Frederick asked Sophie what to do with the money. She told him to establish the endowment. She didn't want the money."

James shook his head.

"How did my mother know?"

"Frederick said she followed him home one Sunday. She saw Laynie and Sophie and put everything together. I guess he admitted everything to her. She kept it secret from everyone for nearly 50 years."

"I can see my mother doing that. She had a big heart and a soul that was as pure as gold," James replied.

"Yeah, I would never have guessed she knew anything," Jason agreed.

"How do we find my sister?" James asked.

"Dad, let's wait until the wedding's over. We owe that to Jane. We'll find Sophie - just not today."

"Okay. It's your day, Dan - yours and Jane's."

Jason was reluctant to tell his father about Bruno. He decided to wait until Dan and Jane had left on their honeymoon. It had been an eventful morning.

"I think I'll ask Jane about Bruno," Dan commented.

"I wouldn't do that. Let her have the day. Don't bring up work," Jason suggested.

"I hate to be gone these next few days with the arraignment and everything happening related to Frederick, Sophie, and the baby."

"Dan, we can hold the fort while you're gone. Besides, I don't think there's much more to do. The only thing left is finding Sophie."

"I don't know. I just have a feeling there's more to this," Dan replied.

"It'll wait. At least for the next four or five days."

Jason stopped at the lobby and let Dan out. He agreed to pick him up in four hours for the wedding.

"We're still going to the cemetery with you and Halie tomorrow. Is your dad going?"

"Yes; we'll pick you guys up at 11:00 a.m. Is that enough time for your wedding night?" Jason laughed.

"No, but we'll make it work."

Melinda and Kenny helped Halie pick up the trash from the party the night before. Jeff left to go home and get ready for the wedding. When Jason arrived home, Kenny was out in the garage, looking at his new car.

"Nice ride," Jason called out as he got out of his car.

"Yeah. I'm still not sure you should be doing this," Kenny replied.

"Hey, with a woman who looks like Melinda, you need a good ride. This car's perfect. I can see you both in it."

"Well, after the wedding, I think I'm going to see if I can get it started."

Chapter Seventy-Two

Linda Phister, Jane's best friend from Wilmington, had come to Chicago to be the Maid of Honor. She stayed with Jane at Dan's house to help her get ready. Now married to a local Wilmington attorney, Linda had turned her life around. The memories of Robert Hollis and Leonard Simpson were distant and unwelcome. She was happy. She felt a deep sense of loyalty to her best friend Jane, who had stuck by her throughout the ordeal.

"Where are Dan's relatives staying?" Linda asked.

"They're all at the Marriott downtown. I saw them Thursday night. They're quite a group. I guess Dan was the eldest and took care of all his siblings. He had a very difficult childhood. They couldn't be happier for him."

"That's really great. I'm sure he would have loved having Alyssa here for the wedding. Remember when she tried setting you up with him, and I spoke up that I'd go out with him? What happened?"

"Guess I got there first - sorry," Jane laughed.

"You look so beautiful," Linda said looking at her.

Jane wore a short, white wedding dress with a simple veil.

"How do you do it? You have the body of a 30 year-old. Only a young person, or you, could wear that dress. You look amazing. I love the shoes you picked out."

"Thanks. I hope Dan likes it."

"Trust me. He will."

Victoria made sure everything was perfect for the wedding. She planned down to the last detail. It was her way of telling Dan how much he and Alyssa meant to them. She smiled as she scanned the crowd. Everyone in her life was there. All of Dan and Jane's family and friends had arrived and taken seats. The last attendees to arrive were Meredith and Michael. As she watched her youngest daughter find a seat, she thought about how much she had changed. The librarian look that Meredith had patented was gone. Now she projected a glamorous image. She walked with an air of confidence and self-assuredness. Soon she would be moving back to Chicago and joining a prestigious medical practice. Michael, her date, was a stylish dresser. His choice of clothing, hotels, and cars spoke of money. Yet, he had no visible means of support. Victoria was worried about her daughter. Only the beginning of the wedding march interrupted her train of thought.

It was a short wedding ceremony. Jane and Dan preferred to spend more time visiting with friends and family at the reception. The outdoor ceremony included a short poem that Alyssa had written, when she was in eighth grade.

On the opposite side of the grounds, around the Conrad mansion, a tent had been erected that included a dance floor. An eight-piece band began playing as attendees began to approach. Jane and Dan shared the first dance. Soon others joined them. Halie and Jason, Melinda and Kenny, and Claire and Jackson were the first to join in. James, at Victoria's urging, agreed to dance as well. As he danced with Jane, Dan thought about his daughter.

"God, I wish Alyssa were here right now," he said.

"She is, sweetheart," Jane replied, pointing to his heart. "She always will be."

"I remember when she mentioned setting us up. She missed on several set-ups, so I was a little reluctant."

"Dan, we weren't set up. We just met and fell in love," Jane said smiling.

Jason too, thought of Alyssa. Halie knew it and gave him moments alone that he needed.

"You okay?" she asked, kissing him on the cheek.

"I'm fine. Just thinking."

"She's here, trust me. She's all around us. I'm sure she's happy."

"I know. I wish she could've been here to see her dad so happy. She really wanted him to find someone," Jason replied.

"Well, he did. She was responsible."

"True," Jason replied, as he led Halie out on to the dance floor.

Meredith and Michael joined the group in a slow dance.

"May I cut in for just a second?" Jeff asked Michael, after tapping him on the shoulder.

"Sure," Michael said reluctantly.

"Meredith, I just wanted to tell you how beautiful you look today. There's something different about you. It becomes you," Jeff told her.

"Thanks, Jeff. Maybe it's that guy over there," she replied, pointing to Michael.

"Maybe. I don't know, but, whatever it is, you're the one responsible. Don't ever think someone else makes you more or less of a person. I'm proud of you."

Meredith sensed something different in Jeff as well. She also sensed that he had deeper feelings for her than she'd known. Looking around the dance floor as she danced, she spied Michael. He was dancing with Melinda.

"Hey, I hate to talk shop, but what's the next step in the Savuzzo case?" Jason asked Dan, as they sat at an unoccupied table.

"Well, after they're arraigned, they'll have a bail hearing to determine if bail will be granted, and if so, how much."

"Think they'll get bail?"

"Al will, I think, because of his medical condition. I'm not sure on Anthony, but I would guess yes," Dan conjectured.

The case against the Savuzzos was strong. Bruno Caseo's testimony and written documentation made conviction almost a certainty. It was vital that the DA's office ensure Caseo's safety. They needed his verification of documents and his testimony. If he didn't make it to trial, the case would collapse.

"I'm worried about things connecting back to my family," Jason responded.

Dan worried about the same thing.

"We can't do anything about it right now, so don't worry about it," Dan replied.

"Easier said than done."

"I know. Just do the best you can," Dan responded.

By 10:00 p.m., the reception had ended. Jane and Dan thanked the Conrads and headed to the Four Seasons Hotel in a rented limo. As a wedding present, Jason had secured the same honeymoon suite that he and Alyssa had shared. He'd sent up a bottle of champagne with a note.

Enjoy Every Day Together, and Love Each Other Unconditionally. If You Do, You Will Be Eternally Happy.
Jason and Halie

James watched as everyone left and went about their lives. He grabbed a bottle of scotch from the liquor cabinet and headed to the den. Pouring himself a drink, he began to think back to his life as a child with his mother and father. He tried to understand what made them do what they did. He couldn't. His focus now was on finding his sister. *Perhaps,* he thought to himself, *Oliver's safe-deposit box might lend clues as to who and where she was.* As of yet, he hadn't had any luck finding the box. He now believed that, if Kenny couldn't find it, it might be lost forever.

Chapter Seventy-Three

At 9:00 a.m., Jason was awakened by the sound of a car engine coming from the back of the house. He looked out the back window and could see Kenny's feet coming out from below the Cadillac.

"I'll be damned. He got it started," he said aloud to himself.

Looking around, he couldn't find Halie. He assumed she'd already gotten up. He threw on jeans and a tee shirt and headed downstairs. Halie and Melinda were sitting at the kitchen table, talking.

"Want a cup of coffee?" Halie asked.

"Sure. When did Kenny get the car running?"

"Heck, as soon as we finished having raucous sex, he headed outside," Melinda responded.

"Too much information there, Melinda. Not a good picture."

"Sorry, but he's been out there working on the car since 8:00 a.m. Oh, and I wasn't kidding about the sex," she laughed.

Halie handed Jason a cup of coffee.

"I think I'll go check out how he's doing."

He had an hour before he had to pick up Dan, Jane, and his father.

"Kenny, are you under there somewhere?"

"Yeah. I'm just checking things out. The car is really in good shape. Your grandfather took really good care of it," Kenny replied.

"Yeah, I know. My dad told me that, when he was little, he used to come out to the garage and hang out with Oliver while he worked on the car. He didn't know why, but when he was about six or seven, he restricted him from going anywhere near the car."

Kenny rolled out from under the car.

"Well, this is one fine automobile. You sure you want me to take it?"

"For the last time, yes, and don't ask again."

"I think, with a good wax job, I can bring the paint back. If not, I'll just repaint it. The engine runs like a top. I changed the oil, spark plugs, and all the filters."

"When did you get all this stuff?"

"This morning. I called a guy I found on the Internet yesterday who specializes in cars like this. He had all the parts I needed. I met him early this morning," Kenny answered.

"Kenny, I knew you would give this car the kind of TLC it deserves."

"I called my dad in Boone last night and told him about it. He wants me to drive up the mountain to show him. It's his hobby as well."

"Kind of figured that might be the case," Jason chuckled.

While Kenny and Jason examined the car, Melinda and Halie talked.

"Saw you dancing last night with Michael Grant," Halie commented.

"Yeah, he asked me when Jeff cut in on his dance with Meredith."

"Good dancer?" Halie asked.

"Yeah, but I think he's creepy. I get a really bad vibe from him. I just hope Meredith is careful. I don't trust him. He let his hand fall down to my ass while we were dancing. I swear the guy's a player."

"Well, I don't know why, because Meredith is beautiful, and she's going to do very well in her practice."

"That's one of my worries. She's a great catch. Not only is she hot and has a great career ahead, she's also a Conrad. If you haven't already noticed, Jason's family is extremely well off," Melinda responded.

"It's hard not to notice. I just hope she takes her time and doesn't get hurt."

Jason and Kenny walked in just as Halie finished her thought. Both had been on the ground, looking under the car.

"Hey, guys, you're dirty. Why don't you start getting ready? We have to leave in about an hour," Halie suggested.

"Fine by me," Kenny replied, looking over at Melinda. "Come on babe - let's shower together."

"Eew," Jason replied. "Please keep the shower respectable."

All four laughed and climbed the stairs to get ready. Jason and Halie had agreed to pick up James and head down to the Four Seasons to get Dan and Jane. Kenny and Melinda would use Halie's car and meet them at the cemetery. It was another nice day in Chicago. A light western breeze made the temperature ideal.

James was dressed in a coat and tie. He and Victoria had been to early church. He was standing by the street when Jason drove up.

"Here, Dr. Conrad, I'll get in back," Halie said, as she hopped into the back seat of the car.

"You sure?"

"Yes, we have Dan and Jane yet to pick up," Halie replied.

James was quiet on the drive downtown. Jason could tell he was distracted. The visit to the cemetery and searching for his sister were only part of James's concern. He knew about the Savuzzo indictments and worried where the investigation would end up. In addition, Victoria had talked to him before church about her concern for Meredith. Pressures weighed heavily on his heart and mind.

"There they are," Jason commented, as he pulled up in front of the Four Seasons.

Dan loaded luggage into the trunk. Jason would drop them off at the airport after visiting the cemetery.

"So, you newlyweds have a good time last night?" Jason asked.

"Oh yes, a very good time," Dan replied.

"I'm glad. You deserve it."

"Hi Halie, Dr. Conrad - how's everybody doing this morning?" Jane asked.

"We're doing great Jane," Halie answered, trying to take the pressure off James having to talk.

It was clear he wasn't in the mood. During the drive, Jane gave them an update on what they'd be doing in St. Bart's. Dan's family had already left to return to their homes in other states. Linda would be flying out on the same flight as Dan and Jane. She planned to pick up a connecting flight out of Charlotte to Wilmington.

Melinda and Kenny had already arrived at the cemetery and were standing by Alyssa's grave. Jason and Halie led them up a small hill to where the grave was located. James trailed four or five paces behind. Halfway up the hill, Jane stopped. Coming the other way, leaving the cemetery, was her new boss Lisbeth Williams.

"Lisbeth, is that you?" Jane asked.

"Hi, Jane. Yes, it's me."

"Everyone, this is my new boss, Lisbeth Williams, the Senior ADA."

Dan, Jason, and Halie all said hello and shook hands. Jason looked at Dan. They both had the same thought.

"Jane, I thought you all were off on your honeymoon."

"We leave in a couple hours. We just came by to talk with Dan's daughter."

"Oh yes, I'm sorry. Sorry I missed the wedding yesterday. I had to work."

"That's okay. It was a very nice ceremony," Jane replied. "Do you have someone here?"

"Yes, my mother. I visit every couple of weeks."

"Well, I'll see you at work a week from tomorrow," Jane responded.

As Lisbeth walked away, James turned toward her.

"Morning."

"Morning, sir," she answered.

Dan and Jason lagged behind as Halie, Jane, and James walked up the hill.

"Dan, she looks like the woman in the picture," Jason started.

"I don't know, but she does resemble Laynie Jessup."

"And she was coming down the hill from where Laynie's buried," Jason continued.

"You all coming?" Halie called out.

"We'll be there in a minute," Jason replied.

"Ask Kenny if he noticed where she came from. They were here before us. Don't do it till James is gone. He doesn't need that right now," Dan suggested.

"I'll ask him when we get home."

Everyone gathered around Alyssa's grave.

"Hey, honey. Here before you stands a married man - a very happy man," Dan began.

For the next 30 minutes, they shared news of the wedding, reception, planned honeymoon, and anything that was new in either Dan's or Jason's life. James tugged at Jason's elbow as they began to leave.

"Show me the grave," he whispered.

Jason left the group and took him over to Laynie's grave. Fresh new flowers had joined the ones left by the florist a week before. Jason's mind focused on Lisbeth Williams.

"Here she is, Dad. She died young. Those older flowers are the ones the florist brings every Monday."

"Who brought these?" James asked pointing at the fresh flowers.

"Got me," Jason replied, checking the vase for a card. "No card or name of a florist on them."

"My father bought this plot for her?" James asked.

"Yes, he did."

Chapter Seventy-Four

After dropping James off at home, Jason and Halie took Jane and Dan to the airport. Linda Phister was already there.

"I hate to leave you with all this," Dan started.

"Go have a great honeymoon," Jason replied.

Linda had met Halie at the wedding and stood closeby, talking with her and Jane. They were getting to know each other. Linda had been a big part of Jason's life in Wilmington and now was trying to move forward with a new life.

"Hey, you guys had better get going, or you'll miss your flight," Jason commented.

Dan, Jane, and Linda waved as they walked into the security line.

"They look happy," Halie said, as they walked toward their car.

"I know. They deserve some happiness."

"You and Dan really saved each other. You know that, don't you?" Halie responded.

"What do you mean?"

"You both suffered so much when Alyssa died. I imagine having each other to lean on meant a lot. When you joined the Chicago Police Department, it had to be a happy day for Dan."

"I guess you're right. I never thought of it that way."

By the time they arrived home, Kenny and Melinda had already fixed lunch. Kenny grilled burgers in the back yard, while Melinda made potato salad and set the table on the back porch.

"Hey, we just thought we should do something around here, so we made lunch for you guys," Melinda said, as they came inside the front door.

"That's nice," Halie replied.

"Kenny's on the grill? You sure he can handle that?" Jason asked.

"Oh yeah. You should see him in Boone. He's a master. His dad taught him everything he knows."

The four friends spent the afternoon eating, drinking, and talking. Halie fit into the group with such ease and comfort that it was as if she had always been there.

"You all ready for your interviews tomorrow?" Jason asked.

"I think so. Mine's at 9:00 a.m. and Melinda's is at 1:00 p.m. I should be done in time to take her to her appointment."

"Your dad did a great job. He must have a really good network," Melinda added.

"We'ew interviewing with not only the Program Directors but also several of the faculty and the Hospital CEO. I've never met a Hospital CEO before."

"Yeah, he's done a lot for the medical community. I imagine they'll be pretty receptive. Hey, you guys are the best, so, wherever you go, they're going to be really lucky," Jason commented.

"You gonna drive the car?" Halie asked.

"Actually, yes. I made an appointment with a detailer, and I'm going to take it there after I drop Melinda off. I want to see what he can do in three or four hours."

The gift of the car had meant more than Jason realized. It was something Kenny never imagined he could afford. Jason also felt good about the fact that Oliver's prize possession would be so well cared for.

"I talked to Jeff this morning. After your interviews tomorrow, he's going to meet us at Four Degrees for happy hour and dinner," Jason informed them.

"What is Four Degrees?" Melinda asked.

"It's a restaurant and bar that Jeff partially owns. Halie and I went there on one of our first dates. I think Jeff likes to show it off."

"That should be fun. By then, we'll be ready to blow off some steam," Kenny replied.

"So, what's the attire?" Melinda asked. "I don't want to get in trouble again. I guess I was a little over the top at the party."

"You had a top on? I didn't realize that," Jason laughed.

Melinda picked up a piece of toast and tossed it at Jason, barely missing his head.

"Sweetheart, I thought you looked awesome," Kenny said as he reached out for her hand.

"Would you all mind if I borrow Kenny for a little while?" Jason asked.

"Sure - we'll clean up," Melinda replied.

Kenny followed Jason inside.

"Where we going?" Kenny asked.

"My computer. I need your help."

Jason sat down at his laptop and logged in.

"Sit down, Kenny. This may take a little longer than I thought."

He wrote a name on a legal pad and handed it to Kenny.

"Who is Lisbeth Williams?" Kenny asked.

"A Chicago DA. We saw her at the cemetery. Remember? She was the African-American woman we stopped to talk to. You guys were already at the grave. I suspect she's Laynie Jessup's daughter Sophie."

"Okay - what am I supposed to do?"

"I want to know everything possible about her - everything," Jason responded.

"This could take a while."

"That's alright. I'll take the gals to a movie and stop and get pizza to bring home. This is really important, Kenny. Will you do it?"

"Sure, just leave me alone for a while."

Jason went outside and explained to Halie and Melinda what he had asked Kenny to do. They understood and agreed to vacate with him.

"You're paying for the movie and pizza, right?" Melinda laughed.

"Yes, I'll even take you all shopping if it gives Kenny a little more time to work."

"Gonna buy my new dress for tonight, Mr. Moneybags?" Melinda joked.

"Okay, I'll buy each of you a new dress to wear tonight, but I get to approve it - deal?"

"What's the matter Jason? Do you think I'm going to dress like I did at the party again?" Melinda replied.

"Duh, yes. Do we have a deal?"

"We have a deal," she replied.

Halie reached over and kissed him on the cheek.

"Thanks sweetheart. That was nice."

Sitting in the waiting room at Neiman Marcus, Jason wondered if Kenny had been able to come up with anything. It had been four hours. After a movie and drinks, they had reached their final stop. Melinda had tried on six different dresses. Finally, she decided on one that Jason put his seal of approval on. Halie, to his surprise, tried on dresses far more revealing than Melinda's. The last one gave both Jason and Melinda pause. It was a low-cut, tight, white dress that was slit down the side.

"Oh, my God. You look amazing," Melinda said as soon as she saw Halie in the dress.

Halie had taken her hair down. Her red hair set against the white dress drew attention to her face and eyes. Other shoppers stopped to look.

"Baby, I'm speechless. You look so beautiful," Jason commented. "That's the dress for tonight."

"Thanks, babe. I thought Melinda looked great in the one she picked out."

"I looked like chopped liver compared to you," Melinda responded. "I think we know where the eyes in the room will be looking tonight."

The final stop was for pizza. By the time they arrived home, it had been five hours.

"I'm gonna go check on Kenny. That okay?" Jason asked.

"Sure - we'll get the pizza ready and open some wine," Halie replied.

Kenny was still working in the den. He'd printed out a number of pages of information.

"So, any progress?" Jason asked.

"I think so. Sit down, and I'll tell you about Lisbeth Williams."

Chapter Seventy-Five

February 1968

Sophie Jessup took the bus to DePaul University every day. It was a 40-minute ride. It gave her a chance to study before class. She enjoyed the ride. She was 20 years old. She had chosen DePaul because it was close to home and had a good reputation. Since high school, she had wanted to become a lawyer. Her guardians, Frederick Menick and Gertrude Menick, had supported her dream. To them, she was their daughter and granddaughter. They would protect her, no matter what.

Although she was a beautiful woman, she didn't date. She had no time. Walking across campus, she drew stares of admiration from male students. She looked like her mother. A child of mixed race, she had gotten the best physical attributes from each of her parents. Her skin, lighter than her mother's, was smooth and without flaw. Her long, straight hair reached her mid-back. She had her mother's eyes. Asked to numerous fraternity events, parties, and dances, she had always refused. To her, they were a waste of time.

She grew up fast. Watching her mother's short life convinced her not to waste a day. Throughout high school, she excelled, finishing first in her class of 458 students. The academic scholarship she received from DePaul paid her tuition. She chose to live at home instead of on campus, because she wanted to be able to help Gertrude. Frederick lived with Oliver and Miriam Conrad during the week and came home only on Sunday.

Sunday nights were family nights for Sophie. She and Gertrude would make dinner for Frederick and his friend Bruno. The four would sit at the dinner table and tell stories and laugh together. Her mother Laynie and Frederick's sister Rita had been part of the group, until Laynie died in 1957, and Rita, soon thereafter. Since then, Frederick and Bruno had relied on each other.

"Sophie, how's school going?" Frederick asked.

"Good. I'm looking forward to the end of the year. Then, it'll just be one more year to go."

"Then three years of law school, right?" Bruno asked.

"Yes, if I get in."

"Sophie, you're number one in your class at DePaul. Don't worry. You'll get in. You just have to decide where you want to go," Frederick responded.

"I'm going to stay at DePaul. I like it, and they have a good law school."

"What do you want to do after law school?" Gertrude asked.

"I want to be a prosecutor. Hopefully, here in Chicago," she answered.

"Oh great," Bruno chuckled. "Just don't arrest me some day, okay?"

"Uncle B, just make sure you stay clean, and I won't."

Everyone laughed and continued to tell stories. Bruno was a master joke teller and kept them entertained every opportunity he had.

May 1969

Graduation ceremonies at DePaul were held in a large outdoor quadrangle. As the Valedictorian of the class, Sophie gave a short address to her classmates during the ceremony. As a sophomore usher, James Conrad stood in the back. He didn't pay any attention to the speakers. He did wonder who Sophie was. Like his friends, he had seen her around campus and was taken by her beauty. The word had spread that she wasn't interested in dating. Tony had asked her out once but had been rebuked.

Following the ceremony, Sophie, Frederick, Gertrude, and Bruno drove out to the cemetery. Both Laynie and Rita had been buried there. Sophie wanted them to see her in her academic robes. It had been something her mother always wanted her to accomplish. She left her cap on the headstone of her mother's grave when she left.

"I wish she were here to see this," Frederick commented. "She would be so proud."

"I do, too. I miss her," Sophie replied.

"Let's go out to dinner tonight to celebrate," Bruno suggested.

"Well, it is Sunday. I can sleep late tomorrow," Frederick replied.

After stopping at home to change clothes, they ended up at Gene & Georgetti's on Franklin Street at Bruno's suggestion. It was an Italian restaurant famous for attracting celebrities.

"Wow - this is a nice place," Gertrude commented as they stood at the hostess stand.

"Mr. Caseo, it's a pleasure to see you. You'll be dining with us tonight?" the hostess asked.

"Yes, a party of six."

Frederick looked at Bruno with raised eyebrows until he understood what he was doing.

"They know you, Bruno?" Sophie asked.

"Ah, yeah, I've been here a few times."

Bruno had accompanied Lou and Al Savuzzo to the restaurant several times. The owners knew him and made sure he had a good table.

"A toast to Sophie," Bruno said, lifting his glass.

"To Sophie," Frederick added. "May you continue to accomplish your dreams. You deserve all the good things in life."

The empty chairs at the end of the table saddened the evening. Bruno had asked for a table for six. The empty chairs were symbols. They represented how much Rita and Laynie were still part of their lives.

Sophie, now 21, excused herself and walked up to the bar to order a martini. She hadn't ever ordered a drink at a bar. It was a first. Standing at the end of the bar was a young Black man, Ronald Williams.

"You just graduate?" he asked.

"Yes, how did you know?"

"Your table, the celebration, the time of year. It all fits."

"Wow - you're observant."

"Well, I cheated. I also heard the toast."

"Ah, now it comes out. How about you?" Sophie asked.

The young man looked down as if embarrassed.

"Me, too. I just graduated as well."

"From where?"

"Law school at DePaul," he replied.

"You're kidding, I just got accepted there. I start in the fall," Sophie responded.

Chapter Seventy-Six

May 1972

Law school for Sophie meant long nights of study and days sitting in a classroom. For three years, she maintained a rigorous schedule. As she had in college, she stayed at home and commuted back and forth. Every Sunday night, she would gather with her non-traditional family for dinner. The pressures of the week melted under the warmth of those around her.

One thing was different in her schedule now. Every Saturday - and only Saturday night, due to her study schedule - she went out with Ronald Williams. They dated for three years, and, on several occasions, he joined her for Sunday dinner. He was a shy, introverted man with a surprisingly good sense of humor. Few rarely saw it, as he preferred to remain in the background. The nights he spent with Sophie's family, he'd open up.

"You're a funny guy, Ronald," Bruno quipped.

"Thanks, Bruno. That's a lot coming from someone like you. You're the best joke teller I've ever heard."

"Don't get him started again," Gertrude said, as she cleaned plates from the table.

Frederick was pleased that Sophie had found someone like Ronald. He was a good man, with a good heart. Sophie moved into the kitchen to help Gertrude do the dishes. Bruno and Frederick joined Ronald in the living room.

"So, Ronald, what are your plans relative to Sophie?"

"Frederick, she graduates next week, and I'd like your permission to ask her to marry me?" Ronald said, as he pulled a ring from his pocket.

Bruno looked over at Frederick and shrugged his shoulders. Frederick looked back without saying anything.

"Don't look at me - he asked you," Bruno said to Frederick.

"Ronald, you have my blessing, and, I trust, Bruno's and Gertrude's."

Bruno shook his head in the affirmative.

"Thank you, Frederick. I'll make her happy, and I'll make sure she's safe."

"I know you will. Besides, if you don't, you'll have to deal with Bruno. If she says yes - and that's still an if - when do you plan to get married?" Frederick asked.

"I'd like to do it before she starts with the DA's office in September. That way, we can take a honeymoon," Ronald replied.

"That's right. She told me she got an offer last week. She's really looking forward to it. Do you know she intends to go by her middle name at work?"

"Yes, I know. The DA told her Sophie isn't a serious-enough name. He suggested using Elizabeth, but I think Sophie's going to go by "Lisbeth". Sort of a compromise."

"Well, in this house and amongst us, she will remain Sophie - has been and always will be. Wow! Things are moving pretty fast."

"Yes, sir. They have to," Ronald replied.

Ronald had been working at a downtown law firm that specialized in corporate mergers. He was doing well and was being groomed for eventual partnership.

"Then that means probably in July or August. That's pretty quick," Frederick stated.

"I know, but once she starts working, she won't have the time," Ronald replied.

Sophie did say yes and, on August 15th, became Mrs. Sophie Elizabeth Williams. The ceremony was held at Faith Baptist Church, and Silas Thompson, Jr. conducted the service. Sophie and Gertrude had been attending the church ever since Ebenezer Baptist had closed. Silas had met Sophie through her mother when she attended Ebenezer in the '50s. Like his father before him, he had grown fond of them. Not having children of his own, he considered Sophie to be like a daughter.

After a one-week honeymoon in the Catskills, Ronald and Sophie began life in his small home in Lincoln Park. Every Sunday night, they would travel to Cicero for the traditional Sunday family dinner. The death of Gertrude in 1982 devastated Sophie. She had considered her the grandmother she never knew. Frederick still lived with the Conrad family during the week but continued to come home every Sunday morning. He and Bruno looked forward to Sunday dinners with Sophie and Ronald. The sadness they felt looking at the empty chairs that Rita, Laynie, and Gertrude once occupied was balanced by having someone new join their family.

September 1983

A year after Gertrude's death, Sophie gave birth to Gwendolyn Laynie Williams. Sophie had chosen Gertrude's middle name and her mother's given name for the baby's name. The seven pound, eight-ounce little girl was healthy in every respect. Frederick and Bruno stood with Sophie and Ronald when the baby was baptized at Faith Baptist. Gwen became the center of their lives. As Sophie and Ronald became more and more successful in their jobs, they made sure to spend enough time with Gwen so that she would grow up healthy and well adjusted.

Each Sunday, Frederick and Bruno got to watch Gwen grow. From highchair to high school, they watched and participated in her life. Without fail, every Sunday night, everyone gathered for family night. Several times, Silas Thompson, Jr. and his wife would join them. Throughout the years, Frederick would keep Miriam apprised of how they were doing. Oliver never knew. Miriam wanted to make sure that his daughter was safe and well cared for. Frederick, for his part, never divulged anything to Sophie, Bruno, or anyone else about Miriam and what she was doing.

January 2002

Freezing rain fell in Chicago in early January 2002. It was a Tuesday, and Sophie had stayed home to prepare for a case that was to open up the next day. Gwen was in the middle of her sophomore year at Northwestern University. Ronald had spent the day at work. An impending merger had required his presence. The closing was to take place at a bank outside of the downtown loop at 3:00 p.m.

The call came from the Illinois State Police. Ronald had been involved in a car accident on his way to the meeting. A semi had jackknifed on the interstate and had hit four cars coming the other way. By the time Sophie made it to the hospital, Ronald had already died. Grief overwhelmed her and Gwen as they listened to friends and business associates eulogize him. There were no words of condolence that could make them feel better. They had lost the most important person in their lives. Life would never be the same again. Only time would allow them to move forward. Silas Thompson, Jr. tried to console them through his words, but nothing seemed to matter.

"This is so unfair," Frederick said to Bruno, sitting in a pew at the funeral.

"I know. I feel so bad for Sophie and Gwen."

No one noticed the man standing at the rear door, watching. Oliver Conrad left an unsigned note of condolence as he left the church.

Chapter Seventy-Seven

Present Day

"So Lisbeth Williams is Sophie Jessup. I thought she looked like her mother when I saw her at the cemetery," Jason replied to Kenny, after hearing what he found.

"Yeah, she stayed in Chicago after Ronald died in the car accident."

"I wonder why she started going by 'Lisbeth' instead of 'Sophie'?"

"I don't know, but, if I had to guess, somebody at the DA's office long ago suggested it sounded more professional. 'Sophie' does sound awfully young, as far as names go," Kenny conjectured.

"What happened to her daughter Gwen?" Jason asked.

"That's another coincidence that's hard to believe," Kenny replied, as he worked on the computer to pull up information.

Before long he turned the monitor towards Jason.

"Gwen Williams - your cousin, I believe. Would she be your cousin?"

Jason looked at the monitor. It was a picture of brokers who worked for the same firm as his friend, Jeff Dodson. In the upper left corner was a picture of Jeff, and, in the lower right, one of Gwen.

"You're kidding. She's a broker in the same firm as Jeff?"

"Yeah. Maybe he knows her."

Jason sat back, shaking his head.

"Let's go join the girls. It's been a while."

"You going to tell James and Dan?"

"I'll wait till Dan gets back to tell them."

Jason and Kenny joined Halie and Melinda on the front porch. It had been a long day, full of revelations. The mystery of Laynie and Sophie had been solved. Yet, still in the back of Jason's mind was a nagging feeling that there was more that hadn't come out.

Sleep was difficult again for Jason. Too many things cluttered his mind. It was 4:00 a.m. when he finally dozed off. At 6:00 a.m., his alarm clock went off. He had to be at the precinct by 8:00 a.m. He wanted to run by Cook County to check on Frederick before he went to work.

"Hey, you didn't sleep much last night," Halie said, turning over and reaching out for him.

"No, I had too much on my mind. Hope I didn't keep you awake."

"No, I slept like a log. Can I do anything for you?"

"I'll be fine. Could use some coffee, though," he replied.

Halie got up, put on a robe, and walked down the stairs to the kitchen while Jason showered and dressed. Melinda and Kenny were already up and ready to go to their interviews.

"Wow - you guys are early."

"Yeah, we're both nervous. We couldn't sleep so we just decided to get ready and do some studying," Melinda replied. "Coffee's hot."

"Where's Kenny?"

Melinda pointed to the window. Kenny was outside, working on the car.

"I'll be glad when everything gets done to the car that needs done, and I get him back," Melinda chuckled.

By 6:30 a.m., Jason was downstairs and ready to go.

"Hey, good luck today, Melinda. I expect tonight we may be celebrating."

"I hope so. I'd love to live in Chicago for a few years."

Halie kissed him goodbye as he left through the back door.

"I'll say goodbye to Kenny on my way out. Love you, babe," he said as he hugged her.

Kenny had the trunk of the car open and was pulling items out that had been stored there for years.

"Good luck, today. As if you need luck," Jason laughed.

"Thanks, Jason."

"Hey - the stuff you found last night? Let's just keep it between us for now. Is that okay?"

"Sure. I'm looking forward to seeing Jeff's restaurant tonight. It should be a blast."

On the way to the hospital, Jason tried to imagine what Oliver must have been thinking when he signed Laynie's death certificate. He couldn't comprehend the amount of guilt he must have felt. To maintain a secret of that magnitude for so long had to affect him emotionally. At the same time, he thought about Frederick Menick and his family. They'd taken a new mother and child into their home and made them a part of their family. It was clear that they'd provided the kind of loving environment that gave Sophie a chance to have a good life.

Frederick was still listed in critical condition. He was in intensive care on the 8th floor of Cook County Hospital. Checking in at the nurse's station, Jason showed his ID and asked to see a list of visitors. The floor nurse printed out a list of those who had been to see him. The procedure at Cook County was for visitors to sign in at the nurse's station. The list was short. Only two names appeared - Lisbeth Williams and Gwen Williams. The nurse informed him that they had each spent the night and had left only moments before Jason's arrival.

"Has he been awake at all?" Jason asked.

"Yes, he's been under sedation, but he's been awake quite a bit."

"Is he out of the woods?"

"That only the doctor can say, but, usually, if you survive the first 24 hours, you have a good chance. He's a pretty hardy old guy."

"May I go in?"

"Sure, just don't upset him. If you do, I'll yank your rear right out of there," she replied.

Jason slid the door open and walked in. Electrical cords leading from Frederick to monitors checked every vital sign. Looking around the room,

Jason remembered what it was like the first time he'd been in a clinical setting while in medical school.

"Hey, Jason, sorry to be a bother," Frederick said in a low voice.

"Frederick, I'm sorry. Did I wake you?"

"No, I was just resting my eyes."

"You had us worried. I'm glad you're still with us."

"I know. I'm surprised I'm still here," he replied.

Jason approached the bed and stood next to him.

"Can I get you anything?"

"No, I'm fine."

"Frederick, I want to thank you for being one of the best people I know," Jason said, as he took a seat next to the bed.

"What do you mean?"

"You and your mother and sister took Laynie and Sophie in when they needed someone. You didn't have to do that, but you did. You took care of them."

"I did what I had to do. They needed help," Frederick replied.

"No, you went further than that. That's what makes you a man others should aspire to be."

"Jason, I'm sorry I kept the truth from you. I was just trying to protect Sophie."

"I know that, Frederick. I've got to tell my dad everything. He deserves to know he has a sister and a niece."

"I take it you verified that Oliver fathered Sophie?"

"Yes, we ran DNA tests on the remains from the trunk and compared them to my dad's. Oliver was the father."

"I guess it's time. I'm so glad the tests you ran verified that Oliver is Sophie's father. I'm so sorry about what I did."

"What do you mean?" Jason asked.

"Putting Oliver's son in the trunk. I just didn't know what to do. If Laynie had known she'd given birth to a dead child, it would've killed her. I couldn't let that happen. I just panicked."

"Why didn't you remove the remains later on?" Jason asked.

"I just never did. I guess the longer it went, I thought it would be riskier to remove them than to leave them there."

"You know, Lisbeth and Gwen have been here all night. They left just before I got here."

"I know. They were worried. Are you going to tell them about Oliver and James?"

Jason had considered what and how to tell them. The news about Sophie's heritage would be hard for them to believe. Only Frederick could verify the truth.

"Frederick, I think that should come from you."

"I know. I'll tell them today."

Jason got up to leave. He needed to get to work.

"Has Bruno been here?" Frederick asked.

"No, they won't let him come."

"What do you mean, won't let him come?" Frederick asked.

"The DA's office. He's told them everything about the Savuzzos. He's the source that the paper talks about. I'm surprised Lisbeth didn't tell you."

"She probably didn't want me to worry, or she figured it was best Bruno told me," Frederick replied.

"He came right over when he heard the ambulance sirens. He wanted to come to the hospital, but they wouldn't let him. He's really worried about you."

"Bruno - what a funny guy. He has six months or less to live, and he's worried about me. I imagine Lisbeth gave him an update."

"Frederick, I'd better go now. I don't want that nurse to toss me out by the ears. You need to rest."

Chapter Seventy-Eight

Now that the mystery of the dead baby had been solved and the parentage established, Jason turned his attentions back to his other cases - official cases. At 11:00 a.m., Kenny called. He'd just finished his interviews.

"Jason, just thought you should know I've just been offered a Cardiology Residency at Northwestern."

"That's great, Kenny. I knew you'd get whatever you wanted. Now, if things go well for Melinda this afternoon, you guys will be moving to The Windy City next summer."

"God, I hope she gets it. I won't take this unless she's here, too. I don't care if I have to move to Podunk, Iowa, as long as we're together."

"Think positive, Kenny. She'll get Cook County. Of all places, my dad has more influence there than anywhere else. You know, a strong network's a good thing."

By the end of the day, both Kenny and Melinda had reported success in their interviews. Kenny had received an offer. The Orthopedic Program Director assured Melinda that she would get one of the three orthopedic positions at Cook County. When Jason arrived after his shift, Halie was pouring them each a glass of wine.

"Hey, you're here in time for the toast," Halie called out, as Jason approached.

"To good friends and great futures. To futures together as partners, lovers, and friends. Congratulations, guys, you deserve this," she toasted.

"Thank you, Halie. Let me do one," Kenny replied.

"To our best friends. May we always be there for each other."

"What more needs to be said?" Jason added. "Now, let's get ready to party."

Halie, Kenny, and Melinda had already dressed. Halie wore the new white dress that Jason had bought her. He had a hard time getting himself to leave the porch. His eyes didn't leave her.

"Let me go change real quick, and we'll head down to Jeff's place. Oh, and Halie - watch out for the guys. They're going to be all over you tonight."

"He's right, Halie. Stick close to us, because they'll be hitting on you," Melinda laughed.

Jason was dressed and ready to go in 20 minutes. They agreed that Kenny would be the designated driver for the night and that he would chauffeur them in the Caddy. He was thrilled to have the opportunity to take it out. The detailer had finished ahead of schedule, and, thanks to Kenny's wax job, the car looked nearly new. Jason and Halie climbed into the back seat, and Melinda rode up front with Kenny.

"You know, I didn't think about it, but this thing doesn't have any current plates," Jason said as they got on the interstate for the trip downtown.

"Oops," Kenny replied. I guess we'll just have to hope your badge gets us out of any tight spots if we get stopped."

"I don't know what good it will do, but we may as well take the chance," Jason responded.

Between the seats in the back of the car was a pull-down console.

"What's this between the seats, Kenny?"

"I don't know, but I would suspect a console to rest your arm on or to hold drinks. I don't know. I haven't gotten that far yet. The back seat is on my agenda for tomorrow. Actually, I didn't know these had a rear console."

Halie moved over close to Jason.

"I can see how this would have been a great car for drive-in movies," she commented.

"Yeah, I imagine a lot of babies could have been conceived on these seats," Melinda replied.

"Ah, not a good thought," Jason answered.

Kenny pulled up to let everyone out at the front door of the restaurant.

"You're not valeting?" Jason asked.

"Are you kidding? No way, no how," Kenny replied.

"Okay, then we'll wait for you right here. I want us all to go in together."

It wasn't long before Kenny arrived. He found a well-protected parking place in the restaurant parking lot.

"Don't worry, Kenny. You can come out and check on your baby throughout the night," Melinda kidded.

"Don't laugh - I will."

Jeff was waiting inside. He had reserved a table for five for 8:30 p.m.

"Let's get some drinks at the bar first. I have a table in the corner over there."

"Sounds great to me," Jason replied.

"Holy crap, Halie! You look drop-dead gorgeous," Jeff said as he led them through the bar. Jason and Melinda could see eyes following Halie. Melinda had been right. Men and women alike turned to look at her. Men with dates, or wives, did it discreetly. Men who were alone were more obvious.

"I feel like a wallflower," Melinda commented.

"Oh, get off of it. They're checking you out too," Jason replied.

Taking seats in the corner, Jeff ordered a bottle of champagne.

"I want to toast to you guys. Jason told me about the interviews," Jeff announced as he poured everyone champagne.

Just as they were finishing the bottle, Halie noticed a woman at the door.

"Jason, isn't that Meredith?"

Jason turned and looked. It was Meredith. She was alone.

"Yeah, just a second."

He got up and walked over to her.

"What are you doing here?"

"Jason, I could ask you the same thing."

"Well, Halie and I are here with Melinda and Kenny to celebrate the success of their interviews. Where's Michael?"

"He had to fly out this morning to London. He's got a presentation to make to a possible investor in his company."

Jason paused.

"Company - what company?"

"He's putting together a new IT web design company. It's pretty innovative and will be really big when it goes public. I can't say much about it. Michael thinks there are some competitors that might try to take the concept public first. It's pretty hush-hush."

"Well, come join us. Jeff is here. Actually this is his place, or at least 15% of it."

Meredith followed him to the table. She wasn't crazy about seeing Melinda again, but it was Jason, and any opportunity to see her brother was worth having to deal with his friends.

"Jeff, can you add one to the reservation?"

"Sure," Jeff responded, seeing Meredith walk up.

Everyone greeted her warmly, especially Melinda.

"Halie, wow! You look great," Meredith said, as she sat down next to her.

"Thanks, Meredith, so do you. When do you have to go back to St. Louis?"

"Tomorrow. I fly out in the morning."

"When do you move here for good?" Halie asked.

"In about six weeks. I'm really looking forward to it."

Jeff sat across the table from Meredith. He tried not to stare. Purposefully, he engaged Kenny in a conversation about the Cadillac. Occasionally, he would look at Meredith and catch her eye. She would nod and smile back. Throughout their time at the bar and at dinner, she focused on texting on her phone. She was distracted.

The evening was full of laughter. As usual, Jeff entertained the group. As soon as dinner was over and before dessert was served, Meredith excused herself. She had an early flight and wanted to get back to the hotel.

"Hey, have a safe flight, big sister," Jason said, as he hugged her.

"Claire's your big sister. I'm your little sister goofball."

"You okay? You seemed really distracted tonight."

"Yeah, I'm fine. I was texting Michael. He needed some help on the wording of a proposal for an investor."

"Oh. Just be careful."

"I will, Jason. I'm a big girl," Meredith said, as she left the restaurant.

Jeff had called a cab and waited outside to make sure she was safe.

"Thanks, Jeff. It was a really nice evening."

"You're welcome. Have a safe flight."

As quickly as she had entered the evening celebration, she had left. Jeff stood outside and watched the cab pull away and disappear in the distance. He felt an emptiness knowing that she was in love with someone else.

Chapter Seventy-Nine

It was past midnight when Jason finally suggested they head home. The restaurant was empty except for a few employees. Everyone except Kenny felt the effects of a night celebrating. Halie had fended off countless advances by men at the bar. She decided that the next time she came to Four Degrees, she would dress more conservatively.

It didn't take her or Melinda long to fall asleep in the car on the way home. Jason, sitting in the back, decided to investigate the pull-down console. Kenny kept an eye on him in the rear-view mirror. It was a full moon. With streetlights, it was easy for Jason to see inside the car.

"What are you doing back there?" Kenny asked.

"Just looking around. Thought I'd try to get this console down."

With a forceful tug the console gave way.

"Hey, Kenny - turn on the interior lights."

Kenny hit the switch that turned on the overhead lights in the car.

"This isn't a console, Kenny. Damn - this is a hidden compartment. My grandfather must have added this after he got the car."

"What's in there?" Kenny asked.

"Give me your phone. Yours puts out more light than mine."

Kenny handed Jason his phone and strained to watch.

"Keep your eyes on the road. We can't afford to get picked up, with no license plates."

"Okay, okay - don't worry. I'll be careful."

The hidden compartment was approximately six inches wide and twelve inches deep. Jason pointed the phone into the compartment. He could see a metal box slightly smaller than the compartment. He reached in and pulled it out. A lock that required a key to open secured it.

"Holy shit, Kenny. You know what I think we just found?"

"Oliver's safe-deposit box?" Kenny replied.

"That's right. I don't think he ever had one in a bank. That's why my father hasn't been able to locate it. "

"Why would Oliver put it in the car?" Kenny asked.

"I don't know. Maybe he didn't want to deal with a bank. Maybe he wanted to keep whatever is in this thing close to him."

"Yeah, but if something happened to him, it would never have been found," Kenny responded.

"I think he knew me or my dad would end up with the car and would eventually find the box. Maybe this is why he made the garage off limits to Dad when he was growing up."

Kenny pulled into the driveway and turned the car off.

"Let's not mention this to anyone yet. Okay, Kenny?"

"Sure. You make the call. How you gonna get it open?"

"I'll take it to a locksmith in the morning."

Halie and Melinda were both asleep. With Halie under one arm and the box under the other, Jason made his way inside. He put the box on the kitchen table as he passed and headed upstairs.

"You gonna be alright getting the Princess upstairs?" Jason asked.

"Oh yeah. We've done this before," Kenny replied.

Jason helped Halie out of her dress and into bed. He pulled the sheet up and kissed her on the forehead. He knew he couldn't sleep. The box had piqued his curiosity. He pulled a beer out of the refrigerator and sat down at the kitchen table. It wasn't long before Kenny joined him.

"Couldn't sleep, either, I see," Kenny said, as he grabbed another beer and sat down at the table.

"No. I was just trying to guess what we might find in there."

"Are you ready to deal with whatever is in there?"

"Yeah. I want to know what the truth is," Jason replied.

"There's no telling what your grandfather put in there."

"I know. He could have been putting things in there up to the day he died."

"Can I go with you when you open it up?"

"Sure. Actually, I was hoping you would. I wish Dan were here."

Over the next two hours, Kenny and Jason consumed a six-pack of beer. It was 3:00 a.m. when they finally headed to bed. Halie barely moved when Jason slid in beside her. Wrapping his arms around her, he kissed the back of her neck.

"I love you, baby," he whispered.

The next day came early, as Jason and Kenny were anxious to get to a locksmith as soon as one opened. When they left at 9:00 a.m., they left a note for Halie and Melinda, telling them where they were going and when they'd return. Neither stirred from their sleep. Jason carried the box under one arm. He called his Precinct to report he'd be gone, doing a follow-up visit and would be in around noon.

"There it is," Kenny said, as he pulled the car up in front of the locksmith.

"Yep. Let's go see what this contains."

Jason looked around the shop as he entered. It was small and barely recognizable from the street. He was surprised that Kenny was able to find it. An old, out-of-date cash register sat at one end of the counter, and locks of every type and variety were strewn anywhere there was an open space. The locksmith had just opened. An average-looking, middle-aged man wearing horn-rimmed glasses approached from behind a counter.

"May I help you?"

"Yes, we need help. We lost the key to this box and need to open it. Can you help us?" Jason asked.

"Let me look."

The locksmith took the box from Jason and began examining the lock.

"This is pretty old," he commented.

"Yeah, can you open it?"

"I think so."

Setting the box down on the counter, he disappeared behind a curtain into a back room.

"I'm sorry. I'm just looking for the tool I need," he called out.

"That's okay. Take your time." Jason answered.

After what seemed to them to be hours, he reappeared. In his hands was a long, pointed device.

"This is what I need," he said, shaking his head.

"What is it?" Kenny asked.

"A Yale Pump. We use it to open Yale locks."

They watched as he inserted the Pump into the lock and started pounding on it with a hammer. Suddenly the locking mechanism gave way. It was open. The locksmith handed the box to Jason.

"Kenny, can you pay him? I'll wait outside."

Jason took the box out to the car and waited for Kenny. After paying, Kenny walked out of the shop and got into the driver's side of the front seat.

"You ready to do this?" he asked.

"Absolutely."

Chapter Eighty

The arraignment of Alphonse and Anthony Savuzzo started at 9:00 a.m. Representing the state was Lisbeth Williams. Their long-time attorney, Broderick Evans, represented the Savuzzos. Evans was known for representing less-than-reputable clients. Although the Savuzzo family had been the target of numerous state, federal, and local investigations, nothing had ever stuck. Every time it got close, a witness would disappear or back out of testifying. Never had the DA's office had a witness like Bruno Caseo. Not only did he have 60 years of knowledge, but he also didn't fear death. He knew his days were numbered. He wanted to make amends for his transgressions in any way he could.

The state asked for no bail. The judge, after reviewing the case, set bail at three million dollars for each defendant. The Savuzzos met bail in 15 minutes. It wasn't a surprise, nor was it unexpected. The case was set for trial in three months. During that time, each side would be able to use discovery to uncover facts about the case. It would also be a time when the defendants would uncover the basis for the indictments. Bruno's name would come out. It would be the DA's office, along with the Chicago Police Department's, job to protect him and make sure he made it to trial. Lisbeth Williams knew the bigger question was whether he'd survive the cancer long enough to testify.

Bruno hadn't told Frederick that he was going to approach Sophie with his information. When she got the call, it was a total surprise. Over the years, each had kept their work lives private. Each knew they operated on different sides of the law. Desire to maintain their family closeness overrode any conflicts. Sunday dinners never included discussions about work. The one comment that Bruno made jokingly to Sophie before she entered law school was the only time that his employment was mentioned.

Sophie finished the hearing and went directly to the hospital. She wanted to check on Frederick's condition.

"Hey, big guy. How are you feeling?" she said, as she entered the room.

"Much better. Gwen just left. She was on her lunch hour."

"Good. Anyone else come by?"

Frederick didn't think it was time to tell Sophie about Jason Conrad.

"Hey, I need to ask you a question."

"Sure, go ahead."

"What's going on with Bruno and the Savuzzos? I read in the paper they've been indicted. Did Bruno have anything to do with that?" Frederick asked.

Sophie knew she had to tell him what was happening. She hoped Bruno had, but the security around him was so tight that visits to the hospital were not allowed. Over the next 30 minutes, Sophie gave Frederick a rundown of what the case involved and the part that Bruno played.

"Is he in danger?"

"Yes. The Savuzzos most likely have a contract out on his life."

"Sophie, you can't put him at risk like that. He's 92 years old."

"Frederick, he insisted. It was his decision. He came to us. I assure you we aren't going to let anything happen to him."

"I'm surprised the District Attorney doesn't take you off the case, since you know Bruno personally."

"I've already talked to him about it. I won't be handling the case beyond the bail hearing. My role is over. He said it would open up too many possible appeals. The new ADA, Jane Moran, will be handling most of the case. I'll be close by, but she'll be the one on record."

"Jane Moran? Can she handle this, if she's so new?"

"Oh yes. She had a great record in her last job. She'll have plenty of time to get up to speed."

Frederick lay back and closed his eyes.

"I'm going to let you sleep, Frederick. You need it. I'll be back tomorrow. That okay?" Sophie asked.

"Sure. Just bring a couple chocolate-chip cookies when you come."

It was Wednesday morning when Sophie called Jane. Jane left a number to get in touch with her if it was important.

"Jane, it's Lisbeth. How's the honeymoon going?"

"It's great. We've spent a lot of time on the beach. It's a beautiful island."

"I'm really sorry to bother you, but I thought I should bring you up to date on a recent development."

"That's okay."

"I think you know about the indictments that came out on Al and Tony Savuzzo. We just completed the arraignment and bail hearing. I'm afraid that when you get back it's going to be your case," Lisbeth explained.

"Really - what happened?

"As it turns out, I know our primary witness pretty well. He's like an uncle to me. I spoke with Josiah. We think it's best that you take the case. We don't want to give the other side any appealable cause."

"When's the trial date?" Jane asked.

"Not for three months. My guess, with continuances, it'll be more like six months. You'll have plenty of time to get ready. All the assets of my office will be at your disposal."

"I appreciate the trust you've place in me, Lisbeth," Jane replied.

"I know it'll be in good hands. I'm available any time you need me."

Jane hung up and turned to Dan. They'd been having lunch at the Eden Rock Resort Restaurant.

"I take it you got the gist of that?" Jane asked.

"You have the Savuzzo case?"

"Yep. That will keep me busy."

"You know, Jane, you're going to have to talk to your boss when you get back."

"Why?"

"Because the source of all the information that the DA's office has is Bruno Caseo. He was Al and Lou's bodyguard. He worked for them for 60 years. James and I talked to him about two weeks ago. I think you may be too close to this. Not because of you, but rather me," Dan responded.

"I think you're right. I'll talk to Lisbeth when I get home."

With two more days left in the honeymoon, both Dan and Jane wondered what was happening back home. Jason hadn't called. Although he knew he wouldn't, Dan wished he would.

"Jane, do you find yourself thinking about what's going on back in Chicago?"

"I'm glad you said that, because, yes, I do. It's not that I'm not having a great time. St. Bart's is beautiful, and being with you is great, but I keep wanting to know the latest."

"What would you say to us going into Gustavia tonight for a romantic dinner and then catching an earlier flight out tomorrow? We can be back in Chicago by mid-afternoon tomorrow."

Jane reached over the table and kissed him.

"You and I think alike. Okay, we have 24 hours left. I say we enjoy the rest of the day on the beach, have dinner in town, and then spend the rest of the time in bed, if you catch my drift."

"Oh, I think I understand," Dan replied.

Chapter Eighty-One

Kenny parked the car in the garage. After closing the garage doors and turning the lights on, Jason set the box on the workbench. They looked at each other.

"You ready?" Jason asked.

"Yep."

Jason pulled off the lock and opened the box. It was full. Oliver had left four 8 by 11 envelopes. Each was labeled. Jason pulled out the first one. Just a name appeared on the front.

Lou

Inside in a plastic bag was an empty vial and syringe. The vial read "Morphine". Oliver had left a written narrative about the events leading up to Lou Sazuzzo's death. According to the note, Al's fingerprints were on the vial and syringe.

"I think this is what scared Al so much," Jason said to Kenny. "See the names of the people this was supposed to go to? He was even going to send it to Al's priest."

The second envelope read.

Equity Partners

Jason pulled out the papers and handed them to Kenny.

"See what you can make of this, Kenny."

After scanning the documents, he knew what Oliver had done.

"This is the paper trail leading back to the Savuzzo family. It's like an accountant's books. It's all here. There are deposit dates, buy-and-sell instructions, dates, and times. Oliver documented it all. He must have been covering his ass."

"Is there enough to convict the Savuzzos?" Jason asked.

"Oh yeah, plenty."

The third envelope made Jason nauseous.

UA-Alyssa

Kenny saw the writing.

"You want me to look at that one?"

"No, I'll be okay," Jason replied, as he pulled the contents out.

Inside were three pictures. The first was of Robert Hollis lying dead in the same ditch that Alyssa had been found in. Clearly, the picture had been taken by the killers to prove he'd been killed. The second picture was of Leonard Simpson, in a similar state, after his execution like murder. The final picture was of a transfer entry in a bank account of 5 million dollars from Robert Hollis's account in the Cayman Islands into a new Cayman account in the name of Anthony Savuzzo.

"What the hell?" Jason said aloud.

"What's wrong?"

"Based on this, the mob killed both Hollis and Simpson. Apparently, before he died Hollis transferred a lot of money to Anthony Savuzzo."

"I always wondered how Anthony could just walk away from all that money that Hollis was stockpiling," Kenny replied. "I guess he didn't."

"I wonder how Oliver got this stuff?" Jason asked.

"Bruno?" Kenny replied.

"I don't know - maybe. He did work there up until two years ago. If Al or Tony had known what he was doing, they'd have killed him."

"Looks like Bruno was starting to make his amends early," Kenny responded.

"What's in the last envelope?"

Jason pulled the final envelope from the box. It had one name on the outside.

Laynie

Inside were three pictures. One was of Laynie, the second, of Sophie, and the third, of Al Savuzzo.

"I don't get it Jason."

"I think I do. Now what Frederick asked me makes sense. I need to go see him."

Jason put the envelopes back in the box.

"We may as well put it back where Oliver hid it," he said, placing it back into the secret compartment in the car.

"What now?" Kenny asked.

"Can you stay here and tell the girls I had to run an errand?"

"Damn. I was hoping you were going to ask me to go with you."

"No. I think I need to talk to Frederick alone," Jason replied.

"I understand."

It was surprising that Jason didn't run any red lights on his trip to the hospital to see Frederick. His mind raced. He couldn't focus. Each envelope contained information that was hard to comprehend. Dan had called and told him that he and Jane would be back in the afternoon. Jason needed his counsel. When he got back, he'd show him the envelopes. Talking to Frederick needed to be done alone.

When he arrived at the hospital, Frederick was awake. Sophie and Gwen had just left. Jason signed in and knocked on the glass. Frederick waved him in.

"How're you this morning, Frederick?"

"Better, I think. Have a cookie. Sophie brought them."

"No, thanks."

"So what brings you by this morning?"

Jason paused. He didn't know how to broach the topic. Frederick's words from his last visit repeated themselves in his mind.

"Frederick, the last time I was here, you said something that I can't get out of my head."

"What?"

"You asked me if we had confirmed that Oliver was Sophie's father."

"I don't understand."

Frederick knew what Jason was driving at. He knew after he made the remark that it had been a mistake. He knew that Jason might question why he asked about Sophie's parentage.

"Why did you ask?" Jason pressed.

Frederick turned his head toward the window and closed his eyes. It all seemed so real again. Thoughts of the day Sophie was born flooded his mind.

March 1948

Laynie lay in bed, nursing her new daughter, Sophie Elizabeth. After taking care of what he had to do in the basement, Frederick came into her room to check on her.

"Are you okay?" he asked.

"I'm fine. So is Sophie. Thank you, Frederick, for all your help. I couldn't have made it without you."

"I'm just glad you're okay and that the baby's healthy," Frederick replied.

Tears started to well up in Laynie's eyes. She lay her head back on the pillow and started to cry.

"What's wrong?"

"Frederick, I wish I knew if Sophie was Oliver's, but I'm not sure."

"What do you mean, not sure?" he responded.

"Please never speak of this again, but something happened at one of Oliver's parties before you came to work for us."

"What? You can trust me. You know that."

Laynie looked at Sophie and kissed her on the forehead.

"It was Oliver's last party," she began. "I still can't get it out of my head."

July 1947

"I think I'll cover her up later," Oliver said aloud to himself, after parking the car back in his garage.

The drive had been good for him. The cool night air was refreshing. Being alone gave him an opportunity to think about things. Hearing Susan Simmons talk about her fear for Molly because of the party was a shock. He hadn't realized the negative impressions that were starting to spread. Driving home, he looked at himself in the rear view mirror and wondered who he'd become.

"Maybe you better straighten up before something bad happens," he said to himself while looking in the mirror.

He was surprised to see Al helping Laynie with the trash. Al wasn't someone to volunteer to help. *That's nice*, he thought to himself - *unexpected, but nice.*

Al Savuzzo knew how to gain someone's trust. Laynie never knew what was going on in his mind. As they reached the back of the garage and deposited the trash bags in the containers, he reached around her from behind and pulled her into him.

"Mr. Savuzzo, please, let me go."

Pressing her up against the outside wall of the garage, he held her face in his hands and kissed her. As she attempted to push him away, he thrust his knee between her legs. Laynie could feel him getting aroused. Forcefully he pressed his thigh into her. She felt the day-old coarseness of his whiskers scraping against her neck.

"Stop, stop," she yelled.

Al didn't stop. He pushed open the back door to the garage. He was a strong man. When he placed his left hand over Laynie's mouth, he held a grip that he wouldn't release.

"Don't struggle - if you do, I'll kill you," Al slurred in her ear.

Laynie went limp in his arms as he dragged her to Oliver's Cadillac. The car top was still down, and the light in the garage was off. He opened the door and forced her into the back seat. Pinning her arms against the back-seat cushion with his left arm, he undressed her with his right.

"Please, don't do this," she pleaded.

He didn't hear her or care.

"You can scream, but no one's going to hear you over the band. Besides, most of the people in there are drunk," Al whispered in her ear.

Laynie could smell his cheap cologne and stale, smoky breath as he moved on top of her. As he entered her, she cried out in pain. The more she resisted, the rougher he got. Finally, she leaned her head back and looked away, closing her eyes. Her mind tried to take her somewhere else, somewhere peaceful and serene. It was quick. Within a few minutes, it was over. Al looked down on the crying Laynie with disdain.

"Get dressed, and keep your mouth shut, if you know what's good for you and for Oliver."

Laynie pulled her dress up and buried her face in the seat cushion. She couldn't move. She didn't want to move. *How can I face Oliver,* she thought to herself.

An hour passed. She fell asleep. It was the tapping on her shoulder and the sound of Oliver's voice that awakened her. She quickly gathered herself. Oliver believed her story about the noise of the party and how she had sought refuge in the car. It was reasonable. Thankfully, they fell asleep before he had an opportunity to ask more questions. Waking before him, she went to her quarters and showered. Not enough soap could clean off the memory of Al Savuzzo. Trying to keep busy, she spent the next several hours cleaning the house. It was good for her. It kept her mind off what had happened.

"I can't ever let him know," she said aloud to herself, as she washed dishes.

She finished cleaning, showered again, and dressed for church. She needed to get away from where the attack had taken place. Her church had become a place of sanctuary. Now, more than ever before, she needed it. She needed to be surrounded by those who cared for her.

March 1948

Frederick listened intently as Laynie finished telling him about the rape. He felt rage as he tried to come to grips with Al's brutality.

"Oh, Laynie. You've carried this burden by yourself too long. We need to report what happened."

"No. Frederick, do you think a colored woman is going to get justice against Al Savuzzo? They'll never believe me. What about Sophie? Al will kill us. I know he will."

"We can't just let this happen and not do anything about it," Frederick replied.

"You swore it would never leave this room," Laynie said to him, as she sat up in bed.

"Are you going to tell Oliver?"

"No, as far as we're concerned, Sophie is his child. I won't be here long anyway. I never want to hear anything said that would put that in doubt."

"I swear it won't come from me, Laynie."

Present Day

By the time he was finished, Frederick was emotionally drained. Jason could see the exhaustion on his face.

"I need to get out of here so you can get some rest," Jason remarked.

"Are you going to tell anyone about this?" Frederick asked.

"I don't know. We have the DNA test results. Sophie's Oliver's child, so there's no need to speak of the rape again."

"Thank you, Jason."

Chapter Eighty-Two

Sitting in his car in the hospital parking lot, Jason tried to rehash in his mind what he'd learned over the past two hours. It was nearly noon. He knew Melinda and Halie would be awake. He needed to get home.

Pulling into his driveway, he tried to imagine what had happened to Laynie in Oliver's car. Kenny was still in the garage.

"Hey, Kenny - girls up?"

"Yeah, they're fixing lunch. How was the visit with Frederick?"

"Eventful, but I can't really talk about it right now. Is that okay?"

"Sure. I think they probably have lunch ready," Kenny replied.

"Go ahead. I just need a minute."

Kenny left the garage and went into the house through the back door. Jason walked over to the car and looked inside. He could sense the struggle that must have taken place there.

"This garage has some bad history. So do you," he said aloud, as if talking with the car.

"Hey, Jason, I expected you to be at work," Halie remarked as he entered the kitchen.

"I ended up taking a personal day today. Since Kenny and Melinda leave tomorrow, I thought it would be nice to hang out. The only thing I have to do is go pick up Dan and Jane around 3:00 p.m."

"I thought they would be getting back tomorrow."

"They moved it up. I think they both miss work. Tuna salad sandwiches - my favorite. How did you know?" Jason asked.

Halie pointed at Melinda.

"I remember those long study sessions. You used to beg me to make tuna sandwiches. I'm surprised you forgot."

"Oh, yeah. I was a little fixated."

After lunch, they planned to head to an early movie before picking up

Dan and Jane. Melinda was unsure that the Cadillac could hold six people, but Kenny quickly assured her that it would.

"Kenny, you still need a license on this thing," Jason told him.

"I know. I can talk my way out of it if we get stopped."

With Kenny and Melinda leaving to drive back to Wilmington in the morning, Jason knew he had to find a new place for the box. He tried to put it out of his mind so he could enjoy their last day in Chicago.

"Kenny, have you all been excused from classes? Driving's going to take a lot longer to get back, especially if you have engine problems."

"Yes, I talked to the Dean. She gave me permission – er, rather us - permission to be a couple days late. I think the school likes being able to brag about getting students into residencies like Northwestern and Cook County. They were pretty understanding."

When the newlyweds appeared at the top of the escalator, Dan's sunburn became readily apparent.

"Dan, get a little burned?" Jason asked.

"It was the beach. Jane wanted to stay longer. I finally got her to leave."

"Yeah, like they believe that," Jane replied. "Thanks for picking us up, guys."

"Well, we have a special ride for you today," Jason explained as they approached the Cadillac.

"Wow - you got it started. Looks great," Dan exclaimed.

Jason looked over at Kenny.

"It's his car now. He fixed it up and made it run again," Jason responded.

Dan wanted to get an update, but hesitated to ask, not knowing what Jason had shared with his friends.

"When do you guys leave?" Jane asked.

"Well, first, the good news. We'll be moving to Chicago next summer," Melinda responded. "Kenny got a residency at Northwestern. I'm pretty sure I have one at Cook County."

"Congratulations. It'll be nice having you all here."

"We leave tomorrow. We're going to drive the Cadillac back. It might take a couple days. I was thinking about stopping in Boone on the way. It's not too far out of the way," Kenny said, as he started the engine.

"Okay, then how about everybody comes to our house tonight? I'll grill steaks. We can catch up. Is that okay, Jane?" Dan asked.

"Sure, it'll be fun."

"It's good by me," Jason replied, as he checked with the others.

Knowing he would see Dan later, Jason decided to leave the box in the car. He knew they would get some time alone when he could show him the contents. Although he worried about his boss seeing everything, he was tired of keeping things from him. Besides, he thought to himself, he needed help figuring it all out.

Halie agreed to bring a salad, and Melinda made an apple pie for dessert. Dan made a quick run to the grocery store and picked up steaks and several bottles of wine. When they parked out front, Dan already had the grill lit. Jane motioned everyone to the back yard.

"Jane, tell us about the honeymoon," Halie asked.

"While Jane tells you guys about the honeymoon, I need to visit with Dan for a few minutes. Is that okay?"

Halie and Jane shook their heads in the affirmative.

"Dan, can we go out front?"

"Sure," Dan replied.

Jason led him to the car and asked him to get in the back seat.

"You have me kind of freaked out here. What's up?"

Jason pulled down the back-seat console and pulled out the box.

"What the hell?" Dan exclaimed.

"Oliver's safe-deposit box. It was in the car all along. He never had one at a bank. We found it when we started tinkering with the car," Jason replied.

"Figures. If Kenny can't find something, it must not exist. Now we know why he and your dad couldn't find it."

Jason took the envelopes out and went through the first two. They included items they already knew about. Nothing was a surprise.

"These next two envelopes we need to talk about," Jason said as he took the pictures and bank-transfer papers out of the one labeled, **"UA-Alyssa."**

Dan looked at the pictures of the murdered Robert Hollis and Leonard Simpson.

"Verification of hits," Dan responded.

"Look at the bank-transfer paper."

Dan shook his head as he realized Anthony Savuzzo had gotten Hollis to transfer funds to him before he had Vince kill him.

"Now I know why Vince kept his mouth shut. I bet Anthony used part of this money to buy his silence."

"How could this not have been uncovered?" Jason asked.

"I think everything was about the murders. This wasn't what anybody was looking for."

"I thought UA got the money back."

"They must have missed an account or two," Dan replied.

"We know Vince killed Hollis, but who was used to kill Simpson?" Jason asked.

Dan feared that the picture of Simpson would cause Jason to begin questioning who had carried out the hit.

"I don't know, but it's not really what we're concerned with right now. What's in the last envelope?" Dan asked, trying to deflect attention away from Simpson's murder.

Jason pulled three pictures out of the last envelope.

"Okay - Laynie, Al Savuzzo, and Sophie. What's the significance of these?"

"Dan, I talked to Frederick in the hospital after you left. He said something that made me wonder about Sophie's parentage. After seeing these pictures, I went back to see him again. He opened up. Laynie was raped by Al Savuzzo at one of my grandfather's parties."

"Did Oliver ever know?" Dan asked.

"No, Frederick said no one ever knew. He kept the promise he made to her to keep it quiet. She didn't think anyone would believe her. She was afraid of what Al would do if she reported it."

"Why did he tell you now?"

"I think it had to do with what Bruno's doing. He wanted to release that burden. I also think that finding out that the DNA tests confirmed Oliver as the dead twin's father made him feel safer."

"No chance that Jackson could have made a mistake with the tests?" Dan asked.

"I checked with him again. He told me the dead baby was a Conrad."

Placing the pictures back into the envelope, Dan still wondered why Frederick chose now to talk.

"What did he say about what he did with the dead baby?"

"He said he panicked. He had to act fast. It was the only thing he could think of. I asked him why he didn't remove the baby later. He said he just didn't want to take a chance of getting caught. I also think, although he didn't say it, he couldn't face seeing the remains again."

Jason hadn't let the Simpson picture leave his mind.

"Dan, how do you think my grandfather got all this information?"

"Bruno. Maybe he began to feel guilty about his past and turned to your grandfather. He did say he owed him and respected him. Maybe all this was to keep Laynie and Sophie safe."

Chapter Eighty-Three

The evening lasted until 2:00 a.m. Jason agreed to serve as the designated driver. For Jane, it would be the first night in her married life that she would spend with Dan in her new home. Both of them called their offices to inform them that they would be starting work a day early. Each was anxious to get back.

Jason lingered behind everyone when they got back to the house. He wanted to remove the box before Kenny and Melinda left the next morning. He decided to take it inside and put it under the built-in china cabinet in the dining room. A small cabinet, unused up until then, would serve as the box's new home. Retrieving a lock from the kitchen, he relocked the box and stowed it away.

Kenny and Melinda woke early. They intended to make it to Boone in the same day.

"Hey, thanks for everything, Jason," Kenny said, as he loaded the car.

"My pleasure, Kenny. We look forward to you guys coming back. We need some friends to hang out with."

Melinda and Halie embraced and promised to keep in touch.

"I'll help you find a place to live," Halie said.

"That would be great. I think we'll be moving around June first. Now you guys are coming to graduation, right?"

"Of course," Jason answered. "We haven't been invited to your wedding. I guess you'll have to just send us pictures."

"I invited you," Kenny replied. "You're my best man. Don't you remember?"

"No, Kenny - you never asked."

"Well, consider yourself asked."

"Then, I accept," Jason responded.

The four friends hugged and said goodbye.

"Hey, drive carefully. You're driving something special," Jason called out.

"Trust me - I will," Kenny laughed.

"I'm going to miss them," Halie commented.

"Yeah, I know. It won't be long, and they'll be living here."

Jane got to her office early. She wanted to talk with Lisbeth and explain Dan's connection to Bruno Caseo. Lisbeth had looked forward to turning the Savuzzo case over to her. Waiting for her to arrive, she looked around her office at 30 years of memories. Pictures of Ronald and Gwen adorned her desk and credenza. Plaques given to her by local civic clubs for contributions to the community lined the walls.

"Lisbeth, is this a good time?" Jane asked as she poked her head through the door.

"Sure, come in."

For the next hour, Jane explained her concern about the case. She hadn't wanted to hurt the chances for conviction. Lisbeth listened intently.

"So, let me understand this - Dan interviewed Bruno Caseo?"

"Yes."

"Why?"

Jane explained why Dan and Jason had begun looking into Bruno.

"Jane, Dan's got to file a report. He could lose his job for this."

"I know, but I think he and Jason need to meet with you. Just talk to them, please," Jane replied.

Lisbeth checked her schedule.

"Tell them to be here at 8:00 a.m. tomorrow."

"They'll be here," Jane promised.

As soon as she got back to her office, Jane called Dan.

"Hey, babe, what's up?"

"I just met with Lisbeth like you said. She wants to know why you met with Bruno. You and Jason have to meet with her and tell her why."

"Whoa. I don't know," Dan replied.

"You have to. Tell Jason I made an appointment for you both tomorrow at 8:00 a.m."

"What?"

"That's right, tomorrow morning. I'm not going to let you lose your job for this. It's time she knew some things."

Dan sat back in his chair. He knew she was right. Things had gone on for too long. It was time to talk to Lisbeth both as Oliver's daughter and as the Senior ADA. Careers were at stake. She needed to hear the whole story.

"Okay, you're right. I'll call Jason. We'll be there."

"Thanks, Dan."

As soon as he left Dan's office, Jason headed to the hospital. He was reluctant to agree to meet with Lisbeth Williams, but he knew Dan was right. His mind wasn't on the meeting with Lisbeth. It was on Frederick. He didn't look forward to what he had to tell him. Halie had become his sounding board. When he needed advice, he turned to her. As he approached the hospital, he called her.

"Hey, I need your help."

Halie listened as Jason explained where he was headed and what he had to do.

"Jason, you have no choice. Don't be so hard on yourself."

"Yeah, I know, but it sucks. If I hadn't opened that god-damned trunk, none of this would be happening."

"It's not your fault. You're just seeking the truth," Halie replied.

"So many people are going to get hurt," Jason lamented.

"Stop it. You're doing the right thing. Believe in it and in yourself."

"I love you," Jason replied.

"Hey, I love you, too."

When he arrived at the hospital, Lisbeth was already there. She was visiting and had been called out into the hallway to take a phone call. Jason, standing at Frederick's door could make out the gist of the call. Bruno Caseo had died. The DA's bodyguards had found him. He'd died in his sleep. Lisbeth looked devastated. Her primary witness in the Savuzzo case – and, worse yet, her adopted uncle, had died. Her worst fear had come to fruition. She left without going back into Frederick's room. She never noticed Jason standing by the door. Frederick hadn't seen him, either. As he left by the back stairwell, he wondered what the DA's office would do now.

"Dan, I just left the hospital."

"You talk to Frederick?"

"I never got a chance. When I got there, Sophie, or rather Lisbeth, was talking on the phone with someone. I could hear the conversation."

"And?"

"Bruno's dead. He died in his sleep," Jason reported.

"Oh, crap. That kills their case."

"Not necessarily. If she had what's in those envelopes, could she make a new case against the Savuzzos?" Jason asked.

Dan hesitated to reply. He knew that if the DA had the contents of the envelopes, it most likely would lead to James.

"Hey, where did you put those envelopes, anyway? I hope they're well hidden," Dan responded.

"Oh yeah. I put them under the china cabinet. No one will find them."

"Good. Yes, if the DA had them, the Savuzzos would be history. There isn't any statute of limitations on murder."

Chapter Eighty-Four

Lisbeth arrived at the Caseo apartment at 10:00 a.m. She'd instructed the officers not to remove the body until she got there. Bruno was more than just a witness. He was family. She had never a life without him. He had been there at every turn.

"I can't lose control," she said aloud to herself, as she approached the apartment building. "I've got to stay in control."

Fighting her emotions, she tried in vain to keep from crying. No one knew how close she was to Bruno. Crying in front of her employees would violate her commitment to keep emotion out of the job. A block from the building she pulled over to gather herself. Police cars lined the street in front of the building. An ambulance with its back door open sat by the front door.

"Take me to him," she told her lead officer as she got to the door.

As a teenager, she had visited Bruno's apartment only once. Her mother had made it off limits for fear that Al Savuzzo might show up. Even the interview had taken place at her office. Looking around as she walked to the bedroom, she realized she didn't remember anything about it.

"He went to bed at about midnight last night. Everything seemed normal. He fell asleep watching television," Hansen told her.

"Leave me alone with him for a minute," Lisbeth instructed.

Closing the door, she pulled a desk chair up next to the bed. Slowly, she pulled down the sheet that had been covering his face. Caseo looked at peace. He had died in his sleep.

"Bruno, Bruno, why did you have to do this? Why?" she said, as she touched his face.

Tears fell from her eyes onto the bedsheet. She struggled to keep from breaking down. Her body quivered, and her voice broke, as she spoke softly.

"Uncle B, I'm going to miss you."

Her thoughts weren't on the loss of his testimony and the effect it would have on the case, but rather of the good times she had shared with her overly protective, adopted uncle. Memories of Sunday dinners and non-stop jokes flooded her mind. Taking her chair back to the desk, she noticed that the top drawer to the desk was half open. She pulled it out. Inside, stacked neatly in the front, was a pile of photos. It appeared that Bruno had been looking at them before going to bed. Slowly, she thumbed through the photos. They were all of Laynie, Frederick, Gertrude, Rita, and her as she grew up. She picked up the stack and put them in her purse. Moving back to the head of the bed, she leaned over and kissed him on the forehead.

"Goodbye, my dear friend. Thank you for being in my life."

Driving away from the apartment building, she allowed herself to break down. As she sat in her car on a side street, she cried the tears she'd held back. Moments later, she dialed Gwen's cell phone and asked her to meet her at the hospital. The news of Bruno's death had to be given to Frederick. They were like brothers. It would hit him hard.

Gwen got to the hospital first. She sat in the lobby, wiping away tears, as her mother arrived.

"Mom, can Frederick take this news? I'm worried about his heart."

"We all knew Bruno had only a short time left. The fact that he went in his sleep and not in pain is something we need to be thankful for. I think Frederick will be okay."

Frederick could tell by the looks on their faces that it was bad news. He guessed that it was Bruno.

"Did Bruno die?" he asked.

"Yes, I got the call when I was here this morning. He went to bed last night and never woke from his sleep."

Frederick looked out the window at the passing clouds. He remembered his old friend. The bond that they'd created lasted a lifetime.

"I'm glad he went in his sleep and without pain. He deserved that kind of death."

"Are you going to be okay, Frederick?" Sophie asked.

"Yes. I'll miss him. He loved you both. We would sit and talk for hours about what you were doing. He was very proud of you."

"Did he ever say what he wanted done when he died?" Sophie asked.

"Yes, we both left each other specific instructions. He wants to be buried beside Rita. He bought a plot next to her when she died. He doesn't want any kind of service. I had to twist his arm to agree to a small graveside service just for family."

"Does he have any family?" Gwen asked.

"He had us. We were his family," Frederick replied.

"I'll call the funeral home and make the arrangements," Sophie replied.

Sophie and Gwen stayed with Frederick for another hour. Sophie had to get back to her office to meet with her staff about the loss of Bruno.

"Jane, can you gather everyone? I need to meet with everybody about Bruno Caseo. He died this morning," Lisbeth informed her.

Jane already knew. Jason had called Dan, and he, in turn, had contacted her. The case against the Savuzzos was now in jeopardy. Without Bruno, the testimony of the three merchants would be useless. Lisbeth knew what his death meant.

"Okay, any ideas? I'm sure the word has spread about the death of our key witness," Lisbeth said as she stood at the head of her conference room table.

"Is the case strong enough to get a verdict without Caseo?" a young staff attorney asked.

"With him I gave us an 80-20 shot. Without him it's 10-90," she answered.

"Think they might take a plea?"

"No, they probably already know what happened. Their counsel won't let them take a deal. He knows we're between a rock and a hard place."

Jane, as the new staffer, hesitated to speak.

"Jane, what do you think?" Lisbeth asked.

"Maybe we should withdraw the charges and wait to fight another day."

"You mean give up?" the young staffer asked.

"No, I mean to strategically retreat and regroup," Jane replied. "Maybe we can approach this in a different way and have a better chance for conviction."

Lisbeth walked around the table and stopped at the window. She looked out at passing Chicago traffic and thought about Bruno and Frederick. Suddenly, she turned around and faced her staff.

"We're dropping charges. Jane's right. We need to start this over again. Right now, if we go to court, we lose. I'm not about to lose to the Savuzzos."

"Do you still want to meet with Dan and Jason Conrad?" Jane asked after everyone had left.

"No. What's the use?" Lisbeth replied, as she left the room.

Chapter Eighty-Five

Three days had passed since Bruno had died and since the DA's office had dropped all charges against Al and Anthony Savuzzo. Sophie and Gwen stood over Bruno's grave and listened to Silas Thompson, Jr. recite a prayer. Frederick, who was too ill to attend, would visit the grave when he got out of the hospital.

"I'm so sorry, Sophie. He was a good man. He spent much of his life serving an evil employer. He turned his life around when he met your family."

"Thank you, Silas," Sophie replied.

"Can we go down to grandmother's grave?" Gwen asked.

The short service had ended, and both Sophie and Gwen wanted to stop by Laynie's grave. Silas went with them.

"I brought some new flowers," Sophie commented as she knelt down to place them on the gravesite.

Sitting in lawn chairs four rows away sat Jason and Halie. It was Sunday, and they were making their regular visit to Alyssa's grave. Sophie hadn't seen them. Neither had Silas. Jason watched as they came over the hill and stopped at Laynie's grave.

"Hey, babe: Stay here - I'll be right back."

"Hi, Reverend Thompson, remember me?" Jason asked as he approached Laynie's gravesite.

"Yes, Officer Conrad, right?"

Sophie and Gwen looked at Jason. Neither had ever met him. Sophie knew who he was. She had cancelled an appointment to see him and Dan Johnson three days before.

"Sophie, right? And Gwen?" Jason responded. "My name's Jason Conrad."

"Mr. Conrad, nice to meet you. I think we were supposed to meet a few days ago, but, unfortunately, things didn't work out."

"Yes, I'm sorry about Mr. Caseo."

"Thank you," Sophie replied, as she turned away from him.

"I think you might have met my grandfather, Oliver Conrad?" Jason remarked.

The memory of the day her mother died came rushing back into Sophie's mind. She could see the strange man standing at the door, carrying a medical bag. She was only nine, but few strangers ever visited the Menick home.

"He was a doctor?" she asked.

"Yes, he was. Your mother worked for our family for more than 20 years."

"Really. She never talked about it," Sophie replied, knowing full well that Frederick, too, had worked for the Conrad family.

"I'm surprised you didn't know. Frederick Menick did as well."

"Mr. Conrad, can we do anything for you?" Gwen asked.

"I'm sorry, I didn't mean to interrupt. I just wanted to introduce myself."

"Consider yourself introduced," Gwen replied.

Jason turned around and walked back to Alyssa's grave. Halie had been watching.

"What was that about?"

"That's Sophie, Laynie's daughter. The younger gal is Sophie's daughter, Gwen. The man is Silas Thompson, Jr.," Jason explained.

"The Silas Thompson from the church we found?"

"The same. He lied to Dan and me. He's known Sophie and Laynie all this time. He's been protecting them."

"They're visiting Laynie's grave?" Halie asked.

"Yes, they're here for the service for Bruno Caseo. He's buried in the next section."

Jane had told Halie about having to drop the charges against the

Savuzzo family. The case ended with Bruno's death.

"Jason, she's your aunt, right? Why don't you tell her?"

"Why? Do you think she really wants to know?" he asked.

"Would you?"

"No, but she's going to find out anyway. Maybe I should tell her before she hears anything."

Telling Sophie who her father was seemed to serve no purpose, Jason thought to himself. Once the information in the envelopes that Oliver left came out, they would know. Everyone would know.

Sophie and Gwen waved as they walked down the hill toward their car.

"You know his family," Gwen asked.

"No. Frederick and your grandmother worked for that young man's grandfather back in the '40s and '50s. Actually, Frederick worked there up until the eldest Conrad died of a stroke four-plus years ago."

"You ever meet this Oliver Conrad?"

"Once, on the day my mother died. I was nine, so I don't remember much, but I do remember him coming to the house and checking on her."

Silas Thompson, Jr. felt a sense of guilt as he drove away from the cemetery. He had lied and could justify it only by his desire to protect Sophie. Even at that, he felt compelled to spend an extra amount of time in prayer, asking for forgiveness.

As soon as he and Halie got home, Jason called Dan.

"Dan, guess who we saw at the cemetery today?"

"Not hard to guess - Sophie?"

"Yeah. How did you know?"

"Jane told me the service for Bruno was today. I wanted to come, but she asked me not to."

"Silas was there," Jason commented.

"The minister who denied knowing anything?" Dan asked.

"Yes. I introduced myself to them. They stopped at Laynie's grave."

"How was the reception?" Dan asked.

"Sophie wasn't too pleased. I could tell by her reaction. Silas was feeling a bit guilty."

"Are you going to tell them about Oliver?"

"Yes. When I take the envelope contents to her office, she's going to find out. No way around it. Besides, I think she should know."

"You're going to take Oliver's material in?" Dan asked.

"It's the only way to get a conviction. The material in those envelopes will put Al and Anthony away. Don't you think so?"

"Good chance it will," Dan responded.

As he spoke, Dan kept thinking that it would most likely also put Jason's father in prison. It was something he couldn't let happen. He knew it would destroy Jason. At the same time, he wondered how Oliver had gotten all the information the envelopes contained.

"It had to be Bruno," he said to himself.

Chapter Eighty-Six

September 1957

"Doc, wait up," Bruno called out as Oliver started to get in his car.

"Yeah, Bruno - what do you want?"

"Can you meet me at the Water Tower downtown tonight around 8? I need to talk to you."

Laynie had died six weeks before. The pain of her death touched both men. Oliver dealt with guilt, Bruno with lost opportunity. Each mourned her.

"Why would I meet you, Bruno? Do you think I'm stupid?"

"Doc, I'm not going to hurt you or do anything to you. I promise on my mother's grave."

"Is this important?"

"Yes, very."

"Alright, I'll meet you on the lake side of the Tower."

Driving home, Oliver had no idea what Bruno wanted. They had never spoken more than a few words to each other. Usually Bruno was with Al or Lou. His ominous presence had intimidated Oliver on numerous occasions. The memory of watching him set fire to his car was still fresh in his memory. He didn't consider Caseo a friend. Yet, for some reason, he felt compelled to hear him out.

It was 6:00 p.m. when Oliver got home. Miriam had dinner waiting on the dining-room table. James had brought home several papers that he'd done well on in school and was anxious to show his father.

"Thanks, Miriam. It's been a tough day."

"Anything I can help with?" Miriam asked.

"No, but I need to go out for a little while tonight."

James walked around the table and handed the papers to his father.

"Well done, son. I'm proud of you."

James smiled, feeling the positive reinforcement from his father that he craved.

"He's going to make a great doctor, Miriam."

"He'll be great in whatever he chooses to do, Oliver. He's a Conrad," Miriam replied.

Bruno was standing under the Water Tower when Oliver walked up. He parked his car two blocks away. It was hot, even at the late hour. Sweat rolled off Bruno's forehead. His shirt was wet from perspiration. He carried a small briefcase that he clutched tightly.

"Bruno, let's go across the street and get a drink," Oliver said, as he approached.

"Good idea, Doc."

Oliver was still apprehensive about the meeting. He wanted to meet in a public place, somewhere Bruno would be reluctant to do anything.

"Want something to drink?" Oliver asked as he sat at the bar of the Lake Lounge.

"No, I'm fine. I don't want to take too much of your time. I know you have family waiting."

"So what did you want to talk about?"

"Doc, first I want to thank you for saving my life by taking that slug out of me. I never did properly thank you."

"You're welcome, but you weren't going to die, Bruno. It was a through and through. Nothing vital was hit."

"I still appreciate you coming over to fix me up."

Surely this can't be why he asked to meet, Oliver thought to himself.

"Doc, what I tell you has to stay between us and no one else - agreed?" Bruno asked.

"Agreed. I'll respect your wishes."

"About a year ago, I met someone who changed my life. She is an amazing woman. She has changed me in ways I didn't think possible."

"I'm glad for you, Bruno."

"That's really not why I asked you here, but I need you to understand me. During the time we've been together I've gotten to know her family. I've become part of her family. I had no family until she came into my life. Now, I do. I'm not going to let anything happen to them."

Oliver had no idea who Bruno was talking about. Bruno knew about Oliver's relationship to Laynie and that Frederick still worked for him. He wasn't going to divulge his relationship to the Menick family.

"I still don't understand why I'm here, Bruno?"

Bruno picked up the briefcase from the chair next to him and pulled out a stack of documents. Clearly they were ledgers, account sheets, bank statements, and other assorted papers. He placed them in front of Oliver.

"I want you to keep these for me. Maybe I should say for us."

Oliver began looking through the papers.

"How did you get these?"

"I work in the Savuzzo home. I have for over 10 years. They trust me."

"Why are you doing this?" Oliver asked.

"Because, I saw what you did when you got out of the business. That took guts. I also know you already have some things in that safe-deposit box you told Al about, but I know you don't have enough. I'm going to give you enough to put the Savuzzos away for good."

"Why?"

"Because I have reason to believe they might hurt someone very important to me," he replied.

"Do you just want me to hold these?"

"Yes, and more that I'll get in the future. It's our insurance policy. If we never have to use it, that would be great, but, if we have to, it's there," Bruno responded.

"May I ask who you're protecting?"

"No, just know we - you and I - are protecting those closest to us.

I'll let you know when I have more. We can use this as our meeting place. That okay?"

"Sure, just call this number, and I'll meet you whenever you want." Oliver said, handing Bruno a piece of paper with his private office number.

For the first time, Oliver felt close to Bruno Caseo. The man who had threatened his life, physically assaulted him, and destroyed his property was now in league with him.

"I don't know what to say, Bruno. You know what will happen if the Savuzzos find out what you're doing?"

"Oh yeah. They'll kill me. Doesn't matter, my life's not important. My family is."

"Are you still going to work for Al?"

"I have to. It's the only way I can keep getting information that makes us safe. Besides, what else am I going to do? I've been doing this for so long I don't know anything else I could make a living at."

"You could take this stuff to the authorities right now and put him away."

"True, but that would mean I'd have to go public. It would endanger my family."

Oliver felt sorry for Bruno. Not only had he lost the most important person in his life, he was stuck in an environment he now found repulsive.

"Doc, I'm really sorry for what I did to you. I hope someday you can forgive me."

"Bruno, don't worry about it. Whoever you're protecting would be proud of you."

The meeting had only lasted 30 minutes. Bruno got up and quickly disappeared out a side door. Oliver sat at the bar, thumbing through what he'd been given. Shaking his head, he realized he held Al Savuzzo's fate in his hands.

Oliver pulled his car into the garage. He didn't want Miriam seeing what he was doing. Pulling up the tarp on the Cadillac, he opened the back door and pulled out the metal box he had stowed in a compartment behind the rear console. He'd spent several days installing the hidden compartment. Everything he held on Al Savuzzo was in the box. He told Al it was in a bank safe-deposit box. He took one out that he let lapse soon thereafter. He never wanted the information far from him. He added Bruno's material and closed the box, replacing it in the console. As he covered the car with the tarp, he smiled.

"Funny, the Caddy's my safe-deposit box," he said aloud to himself.

Chapter Eighty-Seven

Present Day

James Conrad knew nothing of the material that his son Jason held. He'd spent the last several weeks trying to find Oliver's safe-deposit box and coming to grips with the idea that he had a sister. He hadn't decided yet if he was going to approach her and tell her who he was. Doing so would open up wounds long since healed.

He'd virtually given up the search for the box. Maybe Bruno was wrong, he concluded - maybe there was no box. He read the paper about the DA's office dropping all charges against his good friend Tony. He was relieved. Sitting in the den, he drifted into sleep. The ring of his cell phone woke him.

"Hey, Jimmy - it's Tony. I guess you saw the paper. All the charges have been dropped."

"I did. Congratulations. I'm sure that was a relief," James answered.

"How about lunch today at the Club?"

"Sure. What time?"

"Will noon work?" Tony asked.

"I'll be there," James answered.

When James arrived, Tony was already seated. As usual, they met in a private room in the very back of the club. Tony stood and greeted his old friend.

"Hey, Jimmy, been a while. How you doing?"

"Alright, I guess. How about you?"

"Good, now that those charges have been dropped. They were all bogus to start with," Tony replied.

"You must have had a leak in your close-knit family," James chuckled.

"That's not funny Jimmy. I think I know who it was."

"So, you still vulnerable?"

"No, the leak is dead. And don't think I had anything to do with it. The guy died of natural causes."

"Did the leak happen to be Bruno Caseo?"

"I'll plead the Fifth on that. I did hear he passed away a week ago. Merely coincidence," Tony responded.

James laughed. He knew Tony. He knew everything that was going on. He always did.

"Ever solve that family mystery you talked about when you came to see Al?"

"Yes, we did. No big deal," James replied. "How is Al, by the way?"

"Not well. We admitted him into Cook County Hospital last night. He's got a bad flu, so we just thought it would be wise. He's got all kinds of stuff wrong with him. I wouldn't be surprised some morning if he just doesn't wake up."

Al Savuzzo had been fighting ill health for several years. Now in his 90s he hadn't left the house for more than a decade. Being wheeled in to his arraignment had taken a toll on him. Now he found himself in the hospital, a place he hated. If the case had gone to trial, just the physical nature of a jury trial would most likely have killed him.

"Jimmy, how are your kids doing?"

"Pretty well. Bill and Claire are practicing here in Chicago. Meredith will start in a month or so with a good group here as well. You know Jason's a cop. He loves his job. They're healthy and happy. That's all I can ask for."

"Any more grandkids?"

"Claire's pregnant. That will make four."

Tony started counting on his fingers.

"You have a ways to go to catch me. I'm up to eight now."

"Tony, you're Catholic, I'm Methodist. You're supposed to double me in that area," James replied.

Even though he hadn't seen him in a good while, Tony sensed that James was doing better. He wasn't as depressed as he was the last time he had seen him.

"Jimmy, you seem happier."

"I guess I am. Everything that's happened over the last few months has changed the way I look at things. I'm enjoying the small stuff more now."

"That's great. Enjoy your grandchildren. Enjoy Victoria," Tony advised.

"I'm going to. I haven't told her yet, but I'm taking her to Aruba for a couple weeks. Just the two of us to get away and enjoy each other."

"Wow, that's romantic."

"How about you, Tony? You gonna be alright?"

"I think so. The worst has passed. I just hope there's nothing else out there. If there is, we'll just have to deal with it."

Anthony knew Bruno was the key to the DA's investigation. His untimely death had been a surprise. Al had wanted to put out a contract on his life. Anthony had refused. He wasn't about to order the death of a 92-year-old man who served his family for 60 years.

"You know, Tony, you could have had Bruno taken out," James said.

"No, I don't do that anymore. You may not believe it, but I'm not my father. If I have to go to jail, I will."

James hesitated to ask his next question.

"Tony, did Al order you to befriend me in college?"

"I'm not going to lie, Jimmy. Yes, he did."

"So, are we really friends?"

"Jimmy, we're best friends. We moved beyond my father's control long ago."

Tony's words were reassuring. James didn't want to lose his friend. He had never believed - even after learning about Al's instructions - that it wasn't a true friendship.

Chapter Eighty-Eight

Ever since he'd heard Jason's plans to take the contents of the box to Lisbeth Williams, Dan had struggled with himself. He was torn between loyalty to Jason, the truth, desire to see the Savuzzos in prison, and concern for the Conrad family. He considered the Conrads to be his family. He knew Alyssa would want him to protect them. He was willing to risk everything to do that.

Lying in bed next to Jane, he slowly stroked her hair and kissed her neck. It was past midnight, and they'd spent the evening watching television and enjoying each other's company. News of the DA's office dropping charges against the Savuzzos was still being talked about on the late news television programs. Dan couldn't sleep. He kept thinking about what would happen once everything became public.

As he lay quietly next to Jane, he thought about the information in the envelopes that Jason held. There was no doubt in his mind that the material would lead to convictions. Earlier in the evening, he'd spent time on the Internet, doing research. Something had clicked in his mind when he looked at the pictures in the envelopes. He hadn't mentioned it to Jason for fear that he was wrong.

Sitting in his office the next day, he called Jeff Dodson. Jeff agreed to meet him for lunch near Jeff's office. It was a cloudy, dreary day.

"Thanks, Jeff, I really appreciate your meeting me."

"No problem - it sounded pretty serious."

"It is, but I need to ask you to keep this just between us. Jason can't know."

"He's my best friend. You can't ask me that," Jeff replied.

"Hear me out. If, when I'm done, you disagree, then we'll tell him together."

"Fair enough," Jeff answered.

Dan proceeded to tell Jeff everything. He detailed the contents of each envelope and what public exposure of the information would mean to Jason and the Conrad family. He told him about Oliver and Laynie and what had happened between Al and Laynie at one of Oliver's parties. He held nothing back. By the time he was finished, Jeff understood. It was hard to believe everything he was hearing.

"Will this stay between us?" Dan asked.

"Yes, but you can't tell Jason I had any part of what you're planning. He'd never forgive me."

"Jeff, I'll take full responsibility. Your name will never get mentioned."

"What do you want me to do?"

"Sophie's daughter Gwen Williams works at your firm."

"She does? I didn't know that," Jeff replied.

"She has for about a year."

"Guess I should have known that."

Dan explained in detail what he needed. It was vital to what he was going to do.

"Can you introduce yourself?" he asked.

"Sure, I'll do it tomorrow. Maybe she'll want to go to lunch."

Pulling out a copy of the firm's picture roster, Dan pointed Gwen out.

"God, she's beautiful. Is she married?"

"No, she isn't."

Gwen was a mixture of her mother and grandmother. She was stunningly beautiful. She had short hair, dark eyes, and a smooth complexion. Running five miles a day had given her a firm, well-conditioned body. Jeff was surprised he hadn't seen her before.

"Wow - she must be on the other floor. I usually know the better-looking women in the firm."

"Rein it in, Jeff. This is serious," Dan reiterated.

"I know. I was just thinking aloud."

"Just keep your focus on what you need to do, okay?" Dan asked.

"I will - you can trust me."

There were 38 stockbrokers in Jeff's firm. Gwen Williams had been with the firm for little over a year. Jeff had never met her. His focus each day was on finding more clients and in doing the best job possible for the clients he had. He rarely talked to anyone other than the two or three people near him. As long as he was one of the firm's best producers, everyone left him alone. It was a surprise when Gwen heard his voice behind her.

"Hi. Do I know you?" Jeff asked

"No, I don't think we've ever met," Gwen replied.

"I'm Jeff Dodson. I've been with the firm for about four years. My office is on the floor below you."

"Oh, I've heard about you, but I rarely get to that floor."

"Nothing bad, I hope."

"No, they call you 'Jumpin Jeff' in the ranks," Gwen answered.

Jeff was taken aback. He hadn't known he had a nickname.

"I don't really understand that name."

"It's a compliment. Actually, anyone who gets a nickname has made it. I don't have one yet," Gwen lamented.

"You will, I'm sure. Why am I 'Jumpin Jeff?"

"Because you seem to jump at every good opportunity. You're, as they say, fearless."

"Hmmm, that sounds good."

"It is. Trust me, it is," she replied.

"Hey, want to grab some lunch?" Jeff asked.

"Sure," Gwen agreed, not knowing why.

Jeff and Gwen walked to Nomi for lunch. It was only three blocks away, and it was a nice day. He arranged for a table at the window looking out over Michigan Avenue.

"I've never eaten here before. It's nice," Gwen remarked.

"They have great food. It's one of my favorite places."

Over the next hour, Jeff got to know Gwen. By the time lunch was over, he found himself genuinely liking her. As she got off on her floor, she turned to him.

"Next time, I buy."

"That's a deal," Jeff replied.

When he got back to his office, he called Dan.

"I got it. I felt kind of guilty taking her to lunch under false pretenses," he told him.

"Sorry, Jeff, but it was necessary. Besides, you need to get to know the people in your firm."

"Yeah, I guess you're right. Hey, Dan, I need to ask for your help when this is all over."

"Does it have to do with Meredith?" Dan asked.

"Yes. Michael Grant, too," Jeff replied.

"I'll be glad to help."

"I contacted Jason and Halie about meeting me tonight like you asked."

"Thanks, Jeff. I know this is hard, but it's right."

Jeff had asked Jason and Halie to join him for drinks at Four Degrees. Dan wanted him to draw them away from the house. Besides, Jeff wanted to talk to them about Meredith.

"When are you meeting them?"

"6:00 p.m. at Four Degrees," Jeff replied.

"Okay, make sure you keep them there for a least two hours. Can you do that?"

"Sure - shouldn't be any problem. I'll call you if they get away any sooner than 8:00 p.m."

"Thanks, Jeff."

It was 6:30 p.m. when Dan walked up to the back of Jason's home. He parked three blocks away so no one would see his car parked out in front of the house. The back door, as he expected, was locked. Taking out a credit card, he slowly began working at the lock until it slipped back into the bolt. The Conrad home was old and the door locks easy to get open. The day before, he'd made up an excuse to come by. He wanted to check what kind of locks were on the back door. The house was quiet. Walking quickly through the kitchen, he entered the dining room. In order to make sure no one saw his silhouette walking by the window, he stooped low to avoid being seen. The small cabinet that Jason had described was easy to find. He opened it, expecting to find the box. It was gone.

"Damn, I'm too late. He must have taken it to the DA already," he said aloud to himself, as he closed the cabinet door and made his way back to the kitchen.

He sat down at the kitchen table to think. Softly, barely audible, he began a conversation with himself.

"Okay, think, you know him. Where would he put it?"

Turning toward the basement door, he smiled.

"It would be symbolic," he said, as he walked over to the door to the basement.

Unlatching the door, he turned on the light switch and walked down the stairs. At the bottom, he looked around for the trunk. He saw it against the far wall under some blankets. Slowly removing the blankets, he saw that the lock had been removed. It didn't surprise him when he opened the top to find the box sitting on the tarp that had been left inside.

"Jason, you're so predictable," Dan whispered.

Before he returned upstairs, he replaced everything as it had been before he arrived. It was 7:30 p.m. Jeff hadn't called, but he knew time was running out. He had to make sure nothing appeared different when they got home. When he reached the top step, his cell phone vibrated.

"Dan, they just left. You have about 15 minutes before they get home," Jeff informed him.

"Thanks, Jeff."

"Get what you needed?"

"Yeah, but it wasn't easy," Dan replied.

Quickly, Dan retraced his steps, being sure to remove any trace that he'd been there. With the box securely under his arm, he walked nonchalantly to his car. He'd parked out of sight but in a spot he could see through a clump of trees when Jason and Halie returned. He didn't want to pass them on the street and give Jason any reason to suspect he'd been there. Ten minutes later, he saw them drive by. It had been close, but he'd accomplished his goal. As he drove home, he felt a sense of relief that he had the box. One final step remained.

Chapter Eighty-Nine

Jane could tell Dan was distressed. His restless nights gave him away. She worried about what he was preoccupied by.

"Dan, are you okay? You seem out of it these last couple days."

"I need to talk to you, but I can't right now. I need to go to the Precinct to see Jason. Can we get together after work at the Kenagly Pub?"

"Sure. You know you can tell me anything," Jane emphasized.

"I know. I'll tell you everything after work."

When Dan arrived at the precinct, Jason was talking to an informant on the phone about a different case. He was focused and effective. Dan was proud of him. He had trained him well. He was a highly effective, well-respected member of the department. As he watched him work, Dan knew he was doing the right thing.

"Hi, Dan. I'll just be a minute," Jason stated.

"Take your time," Dan replied.

When Jason finished, he knocked on Dan's door. Dan waved him in and asked him to close the door.

"Everything alright?" Jason asked.

"Yeah. I just wanted to talk to you for a minute," Dan replied.

"What do you need?"

"Are you sure you want to turn those envelopes over to the DA?"

Jason paused. He had asked himself the same question.

"I have to. The truth's got to come out."

"Okay, I just wanted to check. You and Halie doing well?"

"Yeah she's awesome. I know my love for Alyssa was special, but I think I'm in love again," Jason replied.

"I'm glad for you guys. We going to be getting a wedding invite soon?" Dan asked.

"Maybe - who knows? We'll have to wait and see. But, if we do, you have to promise to be my best man."

"How about Jeff or Kenny?"

"They'll understand. Besides, it takes pressure off them. They can party more."

"I'd be honored, Jason. Right now, I have to go meet Jane."

Dan was going to meet Jane, but only after running an errand. He needed to stop at the hospital.

The fact that Al Savuzzo was in the hospital made Dan's final step that much easier. As a police officer, getting access to the floor Al was on was easy. Thankfully, Anthony hadn't posted any of his men at the door. He never felt like his father was threatened.

"Hi, I'm Dan Johnson, with the Chicago Police Department. I have instructions to look in on Al Savuzzo to make sure he's okay," Dan said to the nurse at the station outside Al's room.

"He's doing well. Probably be out in a couple of days. He just needs some rest and plenty of fluids."

"Would it be alright if I peeked in for a minute?" Dan asked.

The nurse examined the badge once more. She felt reluctant to oblige, but he was a policeman, she thought to herself.

"Well, just don't take too long. He's asleep, and he needs his rest."

"I promise. I'll just be a second."

That's all the time Dan needed. He was on his way out of the hospital five minutes later.

Jason had yet to discover that the box had been stolen. He intended to meet with Lisbeth Williams the next day. She had agreed to a 3:00 p.m. meeting. She pressed him for information as to the subject of the meeting, but Jason avoided the question. Having dinner with Halie, he wondered if he was doing the right thing. Dan had asked him to think about it. He knew the information would open the case back up.

"You okay, Jason? You seem distracted," Halie asked.

"I'm alright. I just have a big meeting with Lisbeth Williams, the

Senior ADA, tomorrow afternoon."

"The same woman you talked to at the cemetery?"

"Yes, same one. She's Jane's boss."

"What're you meeting about?"

"I think I have information that might allow them to reopen the Savuzzo case. Pretty significant information," Jason replied.

"Wow. I'm sure she'll like that."

"I'm not so sure. There's a lot more involved that will come out that I'm not too sure she'll be happy about."

Jason planned to go down to the basement in the morning and get the box. He would keep it with him at work. Only after noticing that the door to the cabinet he'd originally placed the box in kept popping open had he decided to remove it and find another hiding place. Putting it in the trunk, to him, was an ironic twist of fate.

Dan asked Jane to meet him at a pub not far from the Precinct. He needed to tell her what he was doing. He didn't doubt the rightness of his actions, but he knew they were illegal and could cost him his freedom. He wanted to know she supported him. After explaining the situation to her, she reached out and held his hand.

"Dan Johnson, you're a hell of a man. You never cease to amaze me. You put yourself at risk for family and friends without any consideration of what it might do to you."

"I just need to know you'll be there," Dan replied.

"I will be, as will your friends. Alyssa would be prouder of you at this moment than ever before."

"You know I could serve time for this. I've already committed breaking and entering. You gonna visit me in jail?"

Jane laughed.

"I don't think that will happen."

Dan reached over the table and kissed her gently.

By the next afternoon, Samuel Koenig from the Chicago Police Lab had the results. He called Dan.

"Hey, Sam, thanks for doing a rush on this," Dan said, as he entered the lab.

"No problem, Dan. I owed you one."

Samual handed him the results.

"Damn! I was right," Dan said to himself as he looked at the results. "Any chance this could be a mistake?"

"No. None. What you see is factual. I stake my job on it."

"Thanks, Sam, but you don't have to. I'm the one doing that."

"Anything else you need?" Sam asked.

"No - this was exactly what I needed."

Leaving Koenig, Dan drove immediately over to James's house. Victoria told him he was on the way home from a luncheon meeting and would arrive within the hour. Dan decided to wait on the porch.

"Can I get you some lemonade or a soda?" Victoria asked.

"Lemonade would be great."

Victoria brought it out on the porch and handed it him.

"Is everything alright?" she asked.

"It's fine, Victoria. I just need to talk with James for a few minutes."

"Dan, I need to ask for your help," she replied.

"What's wrong, Victoria?"

Tears welled up in her eyes.

"I'm really worried about Meredith. I don't trust this man she's seeing."

"You're not the only one, Victoria. I have a feeling a few others feel the same way," he replied.

"Can you see if you can find out something about him?"

"I already plan to do that. I have a couple things I have to do first, but then I'll start poking my nose around. Is that okay?"

"Thank you, Dan. I knew you would help. Please don't tell James I asked. He thinks she'll grow out of him. He keeps saying she's an adult and needs to make her own mistakes."

"Don't worry - we'll check him out."

As Victoria carried the lemonade glasses into the kitchen, James drove up the front driveway.

"Dan's on the front porch, James," Victoria told him as he walked in the back door.

"I saw him," James answered, as he kissed her on the cheek.

Victoria had noticed a change in her husband. He was more affectionate and attentive. The trip to Aruba that he surprised her with shocked her. She looked forward to leaving in three weeks. It would be a second honeymoon.

"Hi, Dan - what brings you over today?" James asked.

"I need to talk to you about something very serious," Dan responded.

James sat down in the chair next to him.

"Okay, what is it?"

"Jason found Oliver's safe-deposit box."

"Where?" James asked.

"He had a secret compartment in the Cadillac. Jason and Kenny found it."

"Where is it?"

"Jason had it. He plans to tell you about it before he takes it to the DA," Dan replied.

"And now?"

"I stole it out of his house."

"You stole it - why?" James asked.

"Because of what's in it. There's too much that would tie everything back to you."

"I'll take whatever I deserve. I'm not afraid of being exposed," James responded.

"I know, James, but this would destroy Jason."

The truth in Oliver's box would destroy the Conrad family. What

Oliver had done to protect the family ultimately placed it at risk. James knew it.

"How're you going to explain this to Jason?" James asked.

"He plans to take the box to Sophie tomorrow afternoon. He won't find it. As far as I'm concerned, someone in the Savuzzo family got to it first. The information in that box would have led to their conviction. There's no doubt in my mind."

"What else is in there?" James pressed.

"Everything Oliver collected to destroy Lou and Al. It was his insurance policy. James, there also was proof that Simpson was a hit and that Anthony extorted millions of dollars from Hollis before he was killed."

"Tony? I don't believe that. He wouldn't take advantage like that."

"James, he did, and the proof's in the box," Dan responded.

"I want to see the box," James replied..

"No one will ever see the box. I've destroyed everything in it."

James was visibly upset.

"James, I have one more thing I need to tell you," Dan remarked.

"What? You've certainly told me enough."

"Sophie's not your sister," Dan related.

"What're you talking about? Jackson already proved that the DNA of the twin in the basement matched mine. Sophie's the surviving twin - and my half-sister."

"No, she isn't. She's the other twin, but she's not your sister," Dan told him.

"I'm lost here. You'll have to explain," James pleaded.

"Laynie was raped by Al Savuzzo at one of Oliver's parties. You ever hear of the term Superfecundation?" Dan asked.

"Yeah, but I don't buy it. I think it's a myth."

Dan pulled out articles that confirmed it was real and possible. Since 1978, scientists had been able to establish its validity.

"So you believe that Oliver and Al had sex with Laynie close enough in time that two of her eggs were fertilized by sperm from both of them. That the result was fraternal twins with Oliver as the father of the baby that died and Al as Sophie's father."

"It's been proven, James. I researched it. It's not a myth."

"How can you be sure?"

"Well, Jeff Dodson was able to get a hair sample from Gwen, Sophie's daughter, and I got one from Al. I had a friend in the Police Lab test Gwen's DNA with Al's. It's not as conclusive as tissue samples or blood but it was a match. I believe he's her grandfather, and Sophie's his daughter."

James couldn't respond. He had just gotten used to thinking of Sophie as his sister. The idea that both Oliver and Al fathered Laynie's twins was hard to grasp.

"This is another reason I had to destroy the information in that box. I think Oliver knew the truth. I think, somehow, when he saw Sophie, he knew she wasn't his. That's the only explanation that seems possible," Dan explained.

"Dan, please - no one can know this. This would destroy Sophie and her daughter."

"They won't ever know," Dan promised.

Chapter Ninety

Frederick Menick was still in the hospital. He was scheduled to check out the following day. If not for two minor heart issues that had followed his major attack, he would've been home. It was 7:00 a.m., and James stopped by his room to say hello and to see how he was doing. The dozens of wires and monitors that had been there were now gone. He was on the mend and soon would be leaving.

"James Conrad, nice to see you. Haven't seen you since you and Jason stopped by," Frederick said, as James entered the room.

"I'm sorry I haven't been here to see you, Frederick. Please accept my apology."

"Nonsense. No need to apologize. I get to go home tomorrow. I want to go see Bruno."

"I'm surprised you're not on a monitor," James said.

"Oh, it must have fallen off," Frederick replied nervously.

"You look a bit winded. Are you okay?"

"Yes, I just took a walk down the hall. I needed to take care of something."

"Well, your chart looks pretty good. I think you'll have a good recovery. Just don't go having any more heart attacks, okay?"

"I promise, no more."

Leaving Frederick's room, James headed to room 418, Al Savuzzo's room. As he walked, he felt a sense of anticipation. What Dan had told him the night before had made what he needed to do that much clearer.

The elevator stopped on the fourth floor. In his pocket was a syringe containing insulin. Al was a diabetic. He took insulin regularly. Killing Leonard Simpson had been hard. The feel of the pistol going off in his hand and the noise Simpson's skull made when it fractured into pieces had been an experience that changed him, but he felt justified. As a parent protects a child, he considered killing Leonard Simpson to be protecting his family. Now, he didn't find it as difficult.

An attractive young African-American woman stepped on to the elevator as James stepped off. She looked familiar to James, but he couldn't place her. An alarm coming from a patient room could be heard from where he stood. Walking toward Al's room, he checked the hallways. The nurse had left her desk to check on another patient and was slow to respond to the alarm. Looking in, he could see Al's face covered by a pillow. The monitor showed a flat line. Before the nurse and others could arrive, he moved the pillow back under Al's head and left the room. No one noticed as he walked away - just another doctor doing rounds.

As James was visiting with Frederick, Jason was pulling open the trunk. Much to his surprise and dismay, Oliver's box was gone - and with it all the evidence that would convict the Savuzzos and reveal the truth about Sophie's parentage. As he walked up the stairs, his cell phone rang.

"Jason, it's Meredith. I need your help."

About the Author

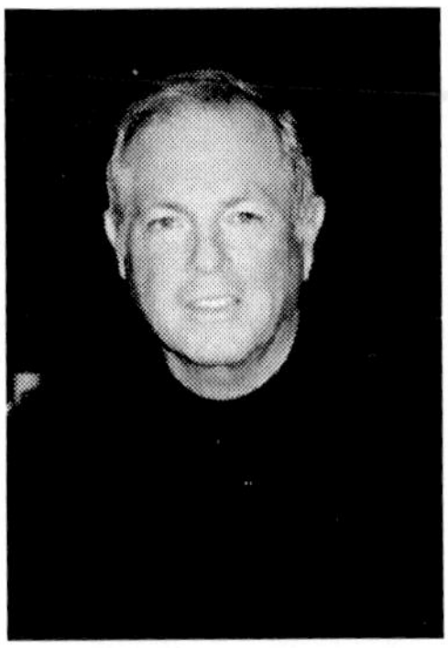

Doug Dalzell graduated from law school in 1975 after serving in the United States Navy. He spent over thirty five years in higher education as a university administrator. The son of a military father he has traveled extensively around the world. Family Secrets follows Seat 23 in the Conrad Chronicles. It delves into the lives of a powerful Chicago family. The novel plays out in the streets and boardrooms of past and present day Chicago. Dalzell, the father of two and grandfather of six, lives in Baltimore, Maryland.